TOM D. NICHOL, D.D.S., M.D.
LARRY D. FLORMAN, M.D.
SUITE 520 DOCTORS OFFICE BLDG.
250 EAST LIBERTY STREET
LOUISVILLE, KENTUCKY 40202

A Woman's Choice

A Woman's Choice
New Options in the Treatment
of Breast Cancer

Mary Spletter

Beacon Press • Boston

Copyright © 1982 by Mary Spletter

Beacon Press books are published under the auspices
of the Unitarian Universalist Association,
25 Beacon Street, Boston, Massachusetts 02108
Published simultaneously in Canada by
Fitzhenry & Whiteside Limited, Toronto

Printed in the United States of America

(hardcover) 9 8 7 6 5 4 3 2 1

Library of Congress Cataloging in Publication Data

Spletter, Mary 1946—
    A woman's choice.
    Bibliography: p.
    Includes index.
    1. Mastectomy—Patients—United States—Biography.
2. Spletter, Mary, 1946— 3. Mammaplasty—
Complications and sequelae. 4. Breast—Cancer.
I. Title
RD667.5.S64   616.99-44906   81-66192
ISBN 0-8070-3258-1   AACR2

To my husband and friend,
Jeffrey Dean Robbins, and to
my mother, Mary E. Knaack

Foreword

As a genetic counselor, I often see women who ask about breast cancer risk—women who have a family history of breast cancer or think they may be at increased risk for some other reason. The women I see want information not merely about their own risk, but also to learn enough about the field so they can frame questions that are important to them. Time and again I have heard women lament, "I only wish I knew enough to know what questions to ask." I have found that women's anxieties about breast cancer are generally the result of too little information, not too much.

Women frequently ask me if there is a book that will help them to learn enough to make informed decisions about their own breast care. They want the latest information, as well as a framework around which to organize and evaluate new information as it becomes available. *A Woman's Choice* is the book many women have been asking for. It presents in clear, concise form a thorough review of current information on breast cancer—from scientific theories and available treatments to the social and personal ramifications of the disease.

A Woman's Choice gives the reader a method for analyzing the most up-to-date findings and enumerates some of the key questions one should ask about each area. Women who do and those who do not have breast cancer will find that the book's approach will help in planning medical care and will find in it an invaluable source of material. Instead of presenting our current understanding as a static entity, Mary Spletter has clarified the uncertainties and explored the experts' disagreements.

Many of the women I see wonder how they would cope with breast cancer—how their friends and relatives would respond, how they themselves would deal with the medical and emotional aspects of this disease. *A Woman's Choice* contains numerous and varied accounts from women who have had breast cancer. By including aspects of others' histories, Mary Spletter has shown different ways of coping and has explored the varied problems that can arise when a woman has breast cancer. By sharing her own experience, she has shown how one young woman has lived (and married) following a Halsted radical mastectomy. She has candidly discussed the tribulations, triumphs, and lessons learned during her search for breast reconstruction. Mary's story is an instructive case history of changing medical capabilities and mores. It is also a deeply personal, warmly human account of one woman's odyssey to learn what she could, and to tell others what she has discovered, so that the passage for those who follow will have fewer uncertainties.

A Woman's Choice will inspire and enlighten many women, whether or not they have breast cancer. Men too, I am sure, can gain valuable insight from reading this book.

Patricia T. Kelly, Ph. D.
Director, Genetic Counseling
Service, Mount Zion
Hospital and Medical
Center, San Francisco

Acknowledgments

I was fortunate in finding many people willing to contribute time in interviews and to share their information and knowledge about this rapidly changing field.

First, I want to thank the many women I interviewed who have had breast cancer and openly discussed their experiences and opinions, as well as those who provided much information and support. Their names are listed on pages 230–231.

My special thanks go to the three key readers who reviewed my early drafts of each chapter and made valuable comments; each is a professional in his or her field whom I chose for their expertise and their belief that people should be allowed to make informed decisions about their own bodies: Gertrude Case Buehring, associate professor in the School of Public Health at the University of California at Berkeley; Patricia T. Kelly, director of genetic counseling at Mount Zion Hospital and Medical Center in San Francisco; and Fred B. Tomlinson, plastic surgeon, Santa Cruz, California.

My thanks also go to Cathy Coleman, oncology nurse, Children's Hospital, San Francisco; Michael Lagios, Department of Pathology, Children's Hospital, San Francisco; and Allen S. Lichter, head, Radiation Oncology Branch, National Cancer Institute, for their valuable assistance in reviewing and commenting on sections of the material.

Contents

A Woman's Choice

CHAPTER 1

My Decision

My own story started in 1972, when I was twenty-five and working at my first job as a reporter for the Milwaukee *Sentinel* in Wisconsin. One day as I was showering, after a workout at a local health spa, my fingers passed over an unusual quarter-sized lump in the upper, outer portion of my left breast. It felt hard and foreign. I suspected immediately that it wasn't a natural or normal part of my body. There wasn't anything like it in the other breast.

But this was before the well-publicized experiences of Shirley Temple, Black, Betty Ford, and Happy Rockefeller. In fact, it was the dark ages of breast cancer. Nobody talked about anything so personal. Magazines did not routinely run self-examination guides.

In all honesty, I didn't consider breast cancer—not even when I discovered the lump. At first, I naively linked it to a recent back sprain. With a freshman-biology-class understanding of human anatomy, I thought my first workout with the weightlifting equipment had forced a muscle out of place. I grew more concerned as discomfort from the sprain disappeared, but I could still feel the hard lump. It even seemed to be getting larger.

Although 1972 doesn't seem that long ago, it was a primitive time for the treatment of breast cancer. When I finally showed the lump to my gynecologist, he did not mention the word *cancer*, saying only that I had "something" that should come out. His wife had had "something similar" and it had turned out to be "nothing," he said reassuringly.

He referred me to a surgeon, who, during my single short appointment told me, "If the lump turns out to be malignant, we will have to remove your breast." It was difficult to continue concentrating on what he was saying, but I know he did not mention the growing controversy over treatment. He told me that if a lump is easy to move with the fingers it is a good sign. This lump was difficult to move, but, he said, because of my age and a negative set of x-rays, chances were slim that the growth would turn out to be malignant.

I asked the surgeon if he could remove the lump first and then discuss my options for further treatment. I hadn't read about this possibility—I hadn't read anything about breast cancer—but I instinctively thought it would be a logical plan of action. He told me that doing what I suggested would be taking too much of a chance. Any residual cells would have extra time to spread, he explained, and if the lump were malignant there might be other microscopic cancers in the breast. Also, he said, it was senseless to be subjected twice to anesthesia.

I was upset for two reasons. First, I had never had surgery in my life, and I was not looking forward to it. And, trivial as it may seem, I didn't want to postpone a vacation to Toronto, Montreal, and Quebec that a friend and I had been looking forward to for months. The trip was supposed to start the following week. The lump didn't appear to be threatening, so I asked the surgeon if he would schedule the operation for after my return from vacation. He hesitated, but said if I promised not to worry about the lump I could take the vacation first. His agreement to delay only reinforced my feeling that I had little to worry about.

During the next few weeks, I found it easy to forget about my lump. We explored the winding cobblestone streets of Quebec, were escorted through the city's outstanding Zoological Gardens and Zoo by a wildlife artist who wanted to practice his English. We indulged ourselves with good food and shopping. I took every opportunity to practice my high school and college French.

In Toronto at a play at the old Royal Alexandra Theatre, I sat in front of a woman who had a horrible cold. I arrived home with her cold, and, instead of going into the hospital as planned, I had to postpone the surgery for another week, and yet another, as the cold moved into my chest, leaving me so hoarse I could hardly talk. During the third week I phoned the surgeon to tell him, in my deepest voice, that I still had a cold. It didn't work; he scheduled the operation for the following Tuesday. I didn't tell anybody why I was going into the hospital, only that I needed some minor surgery.

This was an especially busy time for me. I was working with a section editor on a fall supplement of special stories, fashion news, book reviews, and interviews to appeal to high school and college readers. When I left work I told the editor, "Don't worry; I'll be back in a few days." I had also just signed a lease on a new apartment and hoped the surgery wouldn't limit all my packing.

In the hospital, I reluctantly signed the consent form that gave the surgeon the right to remove my breast should the pathology report show the lump to be cancerous. I had thought earlier about getting a second opinion or refusing to sign the consent form. I wasn't rebelling against having to lose my breast if that was the only way to stop the spread of cancer. I did, however, want to prepare myself for the results. But then I thought, "This is foolish. You've already been reassured that the odds are well in your favor."

I have always been thankful for the one event that foreshadowed what was to come. Since I had been reassured by everyone that I didn't have cancer, I refused to think about what might happen if I did have the disease. The night before my surgery, the resident, who had seemed so happy and easy to talk with that afternoon came back to my room about ten o'clock to get my family's address. In retrospect, I think he had probably seen the suspicious findings of my thermogram, a test I had undergone earlier that day, on which I still had not received a report. But the fact that his eyes suddenly seemed sad, whereas a few hours before we had been joking back and forth, gave me my first indication that my situation could be very serious. I didn't ask why he wanted to know where my family lived. After he left, however, I got out of bed and went into the bathroom to look at my two breasts in the mirror. For the first time, I noticed that the skin was significantly darker around one nipple than the other. A sign of a problem? I didn't know, but I took advantage of the time to say goodbye to my breast in case I would not be seeing it again. I remember looking at it and thinking, "You're really quite beautiful, and I've enjoyed having you as part of me. You know it's nothing personal, but if it comes to a choice between my life and keeping you, you've got to go." A short time to work things out with my body, but I think it made a critical difference in helping me accept the outcome.

The surgeon stopped in for a brief visit before my early morning operation, saying, "In a day or two, you'll be home again." Before surgery, I asked the nurse when I would be back in my room. "If all goes well," she said, "you'll be awake and talking again by two this afternoon."

I remember slowly starting to open my eyes. It felt like trying to lift two fifty-pound weights. I didn't think you could feel like this coming out of minor surgery. The window shades were up, and I could see that it was dark outside. Somebody said, "It's eight P.M." Jeff, the man I had been dating, and the only person I had asked to come to the hospital with me, was beside my bed telling me that he loved me and that my family had arrived from out of the city.

Totally exhausted, I tried to make the pieces fit together, thinking how strange it was and starting to get a little angry because nobody mentioned the operation. I slowly began to understand. I only had enough energy to ask one question that night and I knew there could be only one answer when I forced myself to say, "It didn't work, did it?" What I had yet to learn was that I had had a radical mastectomy. Along with my breast, the surgeon had removed my two chest muscles and some twenty lymph nodes under my arm.

The most important news, however, was that my lymph nodes contained no cancer, which meant that cancer cells had probably not yet begun to spread outside the breast area. Although the growth was ominously large—more than an inch in diameter—my chances for complete recovery were excellent. However, to help guarantee that all cancer cells had been killed, the doctor ordered five weeks of follow-up therapy with radiation.

Looking at the incision wasn't easy. When the doctor changed the dressing in the hospital, he put a towel over my eyes. That scared me more than being able to look at the surgical results. "Why did you do that?" asked the intern who had accompanied him into the room. "Sometimes women have a difficult time looking at the site so soon after surgery," he said. I thought to myself, "It must look awful."

In fact, it did. I looked at it critically for the first time when I was alone preparing to take a bath. I wasn't as shocked by my missing breast as I was by the new appearance of my shoulder area. I wasn't prepared for the hollow and depression under my arm where the surgeon had removed fat, tissue and lymph nodes. I also was surprised to find that the scar ran up over my shoulder and down a few inches into my upper arm.

I remember asking one doctor in the hospital if the hollow under my armpit would ever improve. "What hollow?" was his reply. I knew that I wasn't imagining the new disfigurement and his indirect answer made me wonder if they had lied to me about my positive prognosis. "Would they have told me the truth if things hadn't looked optimistic?" I wondered. However, I reasoned that they would have had to tell somebody the truth, and I knew that neither my mother nor Jeff would be very good at concealing that kind of information from me. I would be able to tell the truth from their actions and what their eyes told me.

My editor hired a replacement to help put the special section together, friends helped move my furniture and boxes into my new apartment and I went back to my hometown of Appleton to recuperate for a month. I enjoyed the home-cooked meals and sleeping uninterrupted for as long as I liked. After the surgery my arm was so weak that I could not hold the telephone receiver for more than a minute. At home, I started to work on the series of exercises recommended to help my arm regain its strength.

It seemed so ironic. I really had felt quite well and healthy with the cancer growing inside my breast. It seemed that all the pain and damage to my body had come from the surgery. Irrationally, I felt I was being treated for the surgery rather than the cancer.

I couldn't wait to buy a new breast form—a prosthesis. In the hospital, a nurse had shown me what one looked like and how to wear it in a bra. The bra was white and lacy but looked like something an elderly woman would wear. I shed a few tears after she left, because the demonstration had forced me to accept the reality of a new body. However, at home, after a month of stuffing cotton into one side of my 34-C bra, I was eager to buy a prosthesis. I knew I wasn't going back to work until I could look normal. There were numerous types of breast forms to choose from. My first choice was a round, rubber form filled with liquid to give it the same feel and weight of a breast. The flesh-colored form fit easily into my bra. A considerable improvement over the cotton, it did a remarkably good job of making me look symmetrical again in my form-fitting sweater. The prosthesis even seemed to move like a normal part of me.

I would be lying if I said that there weren't some bouts with depression ahead of me. Like the majority of breast cancer patients, however, I think my primary feeling was of how much I wanted to live. I realized that being sorry for myself would accomplish nothing; it would be a waste of time and energy. There was nothing I could do to change what had happened.

To my surprise, losing a breast made little difference in my life. I thought seriously about ending my relationship with Jeff, mainly because I didn't know how breast loss would affect a relationship from a man's viewpoint. I also questioned whether he would have reservations about marrying somebody who had cancer—it didn't seem to be a very promising way to start a marriage. And, at that time, I was no longer sure of what I wanted to do with my life, especially since I didn't think I should plan too far into the future. I brought up my reservations. Jeff had firm answers to my first concerns and the last issue was something only I could work through. "I didn't stop loving you because you lost a breast," he said. Once, over dinner, I mentioned that I was thinking of taking an extended vacation, possibly spending several months in Europe. "That's fine, just as long as I'm the first person you call when you get back," he replied.

Because I had known Jeff for four years, I knew it would be impossible for him to hide his true fears or misgivings from me. It was clear that although our relationship could fall apart for other reasons, my mastectomy had not changed either our mutual attraction or our enjoyment of being together. Our relationship might have seemed strange to others, but it fit our priorities and plans. We had met during my senior year in college, but neither of us was ready for marriage when I was graduated in 1969. He had been absorbed in studying for his Ph.D. degree in chemistry at the University of Wisconsin at Madison, and I had been looking forward to my first permanent job as a reporter, a job that would often entail working six days a week on a shift that started at 2:30 P.M. and ended shortly before midnight. On weekends, either Jeff would travel to Milwaukee or I to Madison.

We had plans to marry when Jeff finished graduate school, and our marriage took place on schedule in June 1973, almost a year to the day after my mastectomy. After four years as a newspaper reporter, although I had enjoyed the job, I was ready to try a different phase of journalism. Jeff and I were especially excited about moving West, where he had been offered a postdoctoral research position at the University of California at Berkeley and I a job as science writer and public information representative at the same university.

We adapted easily to our new life in Berkeley, a city just across the bay from San Francisco. Neither of us missed the harsh midwestern winters, and we both seemed to benefit from year-round tennis and jogging.

I loved my job with the university and the chance to write for one of the top schools in the country. There were two other writers on campus, and each of us was responsible for covering particular academic areas. I thought mine were the best: psychology, public health, sociology, some areas of cancer research, and optometry. I could choose an area of interest and look for a story to write. Sometimes the work could be as routine as announcing a guest speaker for a lecture. But, it also could involve helping to schedule a press conference for a newly named Nobel Prize winner, or reporting a new sociological trend or the results of a public health study that would soon be announced for the first time at a scientific meeting or in an academic publication. My job was to translate the material into news stories that could then be mailed to newspapers, radio stations and news magazines. Because the Berkeley campus is such an active place and is in the forefront of research, it wasn't unusual to see material picked up and reported by national and international media as well as by local sources.

When Jeff finished his research position and it was time to decide where our next move would be, there was no question that we both wanted to stay in the Bay Area. Jeff took a research position with a chemical company in nearby Richmond. We bought our first home, a two-story 1909-vintage house that demanded hard work, painting, and gardening. And we had a private party to celebrate my having passed the five-year mark without any recurrence of cancer.

About this time I began seeing reports about breast reconstruction—in the general press and in the professional health journals and magazines that passed through my office. After my original surgery, I had done considerable reading about cancer and discovered early that breast reconstruction was not recommended for women who had had radical mastectomies. By 1977 the articles were no longer so pessimistic. I reasoned that it was one thing to accept a deformity if I had to and another to accept the loss if I didn't.

I was definitely getting tired of my prosthesis. Even though it did an adequate job of making me look symmetrical in my clothes, it was a poor substitute for a breast. I had several kinds. One irritated my skin; another tended to ride up out of my bra. One day, I dressed so hurriedly that I forgot to insert the breast form into my bra. By the time I got to work, I realized something was wrong, put on my coat, and returned home to put myself together again, feeling like the scarecrow in the *Wizard of Oz*. The only thing worse than the prosthesis was the matronly bra it fit into.

In stores, I became aware of the numerous styles of clothes I could not wear comfortably as a result of my surgery. Anything that hinted of a low neckline or was at all sheer stayed on the hanger. When I changed in the women's locker room to go jogging, I could not help thinking occasionally that it would be nice to look like everybody else. Yes, it was time for me to take a closer look at reconstruction. I told myself, "What better way to celebrate passing your five-year survival mark?" When I told the surgeon whom I went to for routine checkups in California that I wanted to investigate reconstruction he gave me the name of a highly regarded plastic surgeon, the head of his department in a San Francisco hospital. My long-awaited appointment turned out to be a disappointment. Gray-haired, well-groomed, sitting in an office that showed the influence of a decorator, this man obviously cared about his appearance and the image he projected to his patients. He gently proceeded to explain to me, however, that he did not like to recommend breast reconstruction. "The results just are not that great. It's mostly for women who live near beaches and want to look better in their sportswear," he said.

His description of a reconstructed breast was of something that would be higher, harder and not a symmetrical match to my other breast. I held a slide up to the light. Admittedly, it wasn't great; there was scarring on the reconstructed breast from the original mastectomy, but it did not look bad either.

The next time I heard breast reconstruction discussed was a few months later at an American Cancer Society meeting on breast cancer in San Francisco. A young plastic surgeon was answering questions about reconstruction. He had several impressive "before and after" pictures of women, one of whom had even been operated on after a radical mastectomy. The results were lovely, if not works of art; I made an appointment with him for the following week.

The plastic surgeon said the procedure would not be difficult. (However, he neglected to tell me that he had never before operated on a breast cancer patient who had received radiation therapy.) He described the same procedure the first plastic surgeon did. He would open the original scar and insert a mound-shaped silicone implant through the incision. To make certain I would be symmetrical, he would slightly reduce and raise my remaining breast.

My husband said he preferred that I not go through with the operation. Yet he knew that the decision should be mine. The procedure sounded so simple, however, that we both finally agreed, "Why not try it?" The answer was soon to come.

I have to admit I was surprised at how happy I was following the operation when I looked at the implant. I suspect that like many "brave" mastectomy patients, I had suppressed how badly I really felt about losing a part of my body. I was disappointed, however, at the way the skin had been stretched so tightly over the implant. It left a lot to be desired and didn't look anything like the pictures I had seen in my plastic surgeon's office.

The surgeon came in soon and pointed out two bluish areas on my skin that he was "worried about."

"Can I throw out my prosthesis?" I asked optimistically.

"No, don't throw it out yet," he said. "Let's wait overnight. If the skin does not improve, we may have to remove the implant."

A few hours later, surgical supplies were delivered to my room. The nurses refused to confirm the obvious indication that the implant was coming out then and there. The plastic surgeon entered the room, said he did not think it was wise to wait, gave me a light anesthetic, and removed the implant. Apparently my initial radiation therapy had injured healthy, normal tissue along with any residual cancer cells that might have been present. Now, stretched over the implant, the skin was unable to develop a new blood supply, and two areas had begun to die.

When I later visited the plastic surgeon, he suggested a new strategy. "You've got to get rid of that badly injured skin," he said. He suggested simply cutting away the injured skin and bringing in and closing the healthy surrounding tissue. "What have you got to lose?" he asked.

I could not believe it. I had lost time from work. My chest area looked worse than ever. At that point, I had an open draining wound where the implant had been removed. There was still risk of infection. At times I had considerable pain. I didn't want to find out what else I could lose. I decided it was time for a second opinion.

The consulting plastic surgeon said he honestly did not think the procedure stood much chance of success. He said there was just not enough skin in the chest area to give me sufficient tissue for a natural-appearing breast. However, he suggested another procedure. Agreeing that I needed new skin, he said he could graft it from the crease where my body joined my leg in the groin area. He would use a microsurgical procedure that also would transfer new arteries and veins needed to provide a good supply of blood to the new tissue. Because the blood vessels are so small, most of the delicate operation would be done with the surgeon looking through a high-powered microscope and using hair-thin instruments to suture the new veins to ones already present.

The negative aspects were that the operation could take as long as twelve hours and microsurgical procedures were known to carry a 15 to 20 percent failure rate. The most common and most serious problem occurred when the vessels weren't successfully joined, resulting in part or even all of the tissue dying for lack of a good blood supply. I also was told that I would have to gain an extra ten pounds. My first reaction was that my situation had gone from bad to terrible. Only a desperate woman or a masochist would go through with this option.

What followed were separate discussions with both plastic surgeons. The doctor who had performed the first attempt at reconstruction said that the microsurgical procedure was experimental and the only option I could choose by which I would lose the old skin, the newly grafted skin, and the implant if it didn't work. Meanwhile, the plastic surgeon I had talked to for a second opinion maintained that the simpler process would not be a good choice because the results just would not resemble a breast. What followed next was depression. I was totally confused and angered by the situation.

I needed to talk to somebody. The doctor I went to for routine follow-up was extremely difficult to reach. When I called him, I was told that all questions on reconstruction should be referred to his nurse. That was fine, except when I called at the suggested time to talk to her, she told me she couldn't talk long because she was busy working with the doctor and his patients. Worse yet, she really didn't seem to understand what procedure I was talking about.

I looked elsewhere for information. I thought of the surgeon who had done my mastectomy. I reasoned that if he routinely did such drastic radicals, he might be able to tell me what luck his patients had had with reconstruction and what techniques they had tried. It seemed logical to consult him since someone had just sent me a newspaper clipping from Milwaukee about women having reconstruction there.

Besides, I thought it would give me a chance to tell him how happy I was that women now have more options about the kind of surgery they want. Since there has been no proof that the radical mastectomy prolongs survival, the trend in recent years has been toward a less deforming, modified radical mastectomy, an operation that does not remove a woman's two chest muscles. There certainly was no question that women with the modified operation have fewer complications with swelling of the arm and with shoulder discomfort. And there could be no question that they would get better results from breast reconstruction.

I placed an evening call to the Midwest. I found that my surgeon still supported the traditional radical mastectomy. As for breast reconstruction, he said he had operated on over 300 women and they "did not seem to need it." He said that although breast reconstruction was being done in a few select cases, his personal opinion was that in my case it would be "doomed to failure."

The more effort I put into making the right decision, the more I realized what a new, controversial, and even experimental field breast reconstruction was. The only thing that was becoming more and more obvious was that it was time to take a break. What I needed was a vacation, a chance to put things back in perspective.

I had never been so sensitive about my appearance as when I was investigating breast reconstruction. I have heard cancer patients explain that when they are in treatment, it is difficult to think about anyone else but themselves. The demands of my job, a three-week trip to England and Ireland, and a night class in human anatomy and physiology helped me break the depression of my first reconstruction failure. (I had to wonder if other women who didn't have my opportunities or who didn't participate in activities would have found it as easy to recover.)

But even with the outside distractions, there were times my sensitivity felt like an open wound, difficult to avoid hurting by the gentlest comments—and few people were trying to put themselves in my position. I asked one consulting plastic surgeon if my procedure would be covered by insurance. "Yes," he assured me. "And if all else fails, we can mail a photograph of you to your insurance company. The way you look, we shouldn't have any problems," he laughed. I didn't appreciate his humor. Admittedly, after my first failed effort, my open chest wound did look awful. I could barely tolerate changing the dressing. But I didn't need confirmation.

Another thoughtless comment came from a second plastic surgeon. "If my wife had had a mastectomy, I would want her to have reconstruction." My new sensitivity made me shudder at the remark, compelling me to question how Jeff could possibly be happy with me and to wonder whether he had married me because he felt sorry for me. I thought, "Is this plastic surgeon being unscrupulous, or is he just insensitive? Does he say that to all his patients? Does he tell women patients who come in to have their noses changed, 'Yes, if my wife had a nose like yours, I would want her to have it fixed.'" If he had to state a personal preference, why couldn't he say, "I think if I were a woman and had had a mastectomy, I would want to have reconstruction."

A year later, with more articles claiming that plastic surgeons were getting excellent results with breast reconstruction, it was time to take another look. I wasn't obsessed so much with reconstruction as I was with trying to understand why my personal experience didn't match what I was reading and hearing about the surgery. And I still wonder whether I would have investigated further if it weren't for the fact that I really didn't want to accept the additional injury to my skin caused by my first failed effort. "It won't hurt to ask just a few more questions," I told myself, especially since I was learning the right questions to ask.

My first step was to phone Netta Grandstaff, then a research psychologist at the Stanford Medical Center, who had impressed me when I had heard her talk in a panel discussion on breast cancer. I knew she specialized in working with mastectomy patients. I also knew that Stanford had received a lot of media attention for its pioneering work with sex-change operations. Rationally or irrationally, I thought perhaps the Stanford staff would be more progressive and supportive of women who just wanted to maintain their natural female sex characteristics. I knew my luck was changing when Grandstaff told me that she was in the midst of setting up a breast reconstruction information service called Images and Options. Similar programs already existed in New York and Washington, D.C., she said.

She was up to date on plastic surgery procedures for breast reconstruction, had seen the results in dozens of women who had been through the surgery, and was sincerely interested in the subject because she herself had had two mastectomies several years earlier. She was the most informed and objective person I had talked to about breast reconstruction. The first thing I wanted to discuss was the state of the art.

Well, she said, three years ago she had had a difficult time understanding why women wanted to have reconstruction because the results were just not that good. Both plastic surgeons and their patients had been disappointed with the outcome. "But since that time," she said, "with improved surgical techniques and more realistic breast implants, I've seen some excellent results. And during the past year and a half, I have not seen a bad result."

My second question: Who was a good candidate for reconstruction? My own opinion was that whether you lost an arm, an eye, or a breast, you should have the most natural replacement possible. Yet, I told her, I was getting the impression that breast reconstruction was only for women who had severe problems accepting life without a breast. It seemed to be acceptable for those who were on the verge of suicide, dressing and undressing in closets, or having obvious sexual or personality disturbances. I just could not rationalize why, to be considered normal and well adjusted, I had to accept looking so abnormal.

But that was the message that I was picking up from physicians and even from the American Cancer Society. For more than four years I had been a member of the Reach to Recovery Program, one of the Cancer Society's most successful volunteer efforts. Through the program, women who already have had a mastectomy contribute time and support by visiting others in the hospital who are just recovering from breast surgery. The intent is to give women information about breast forms and arm exercises, but, more important, to visit them when morale is often low to show them that they can look normal again and continue living full lives after a mastectomy. I found that if I had reconstruction, I would not be able to continue working as a hospital volunteer. It was standard American Cancer Society policy.

The Cancer Society is slow to change, and in this instance, they didn't want satisfied reconstruction volunteers visiting patients because this was still a time when most surgeons who performed mastectomies didn't approve of reconstruction. The volunteers always have been bound by the dictates of a patient's physician. In fact, a woman can't have a visit in a hospital from a volunteer unless her surgeon O.K.'s the visit ahead of time. I suspect that reconstruction also conflicted with the Cancer Society's efforts to show a woman that she was still the same person she had been before the operation. It also was quite obvious that the policy existed because there was serious concern that the volunteer who selected reconstruction had had a difficult time accepting her own breast loss and certainly would not be a good role model for another mastectomy patient..

When I tried to discuss my interest in the surgery with the doctor who had been following me for checkups in California, he asked, "Aren't you happy with your marriage? Is something wrong with your job?" A local newspaper article quoted a surgeon: "Breast reconstruction is only for women with strong self-image problems."

Grandstaff replied immediately, "That's ridiculous. Women who decide to have reconstruction are just as able to function well and handle the fact that they have had breast cancer as those who decide not to have reconstruction. I guess there is just a lot more work to do in reaching people."

Next I wanted to discuss procedures and doctors, about which there was more good news. She told me that at the last major plastic surgery convention she had attended a new procedure had been presented for women who had had radicals, radiation, or who, for whatever reason, needed new tissue in the chest area. The technique involved transferring a back muscle (the latissimus dorsi) and its overlying skin to the chest area. The muscle was actually detached on three sides, lifted from the back and gently swung around to the front of the body. The extra skin that came with the muscle rode over the implant, helping it to resemble a gently drooping and more natural appearing breast. (Without the skin, an implant, as I found, looked like a round firm bowl bulging out from the chest wall.) The back muscle filled in the chest wall where the muscles had been removed in the radical mastectomy. Since the back muscle was still attached to its original blood supply on one side, it wasn't necessary to join old and new vessels as was required in the microsurgical procedure. I was told that the back muscle wouldn't be missed by the body as it wasn't needed for any major activity. Finally, experience in other parts of the country had shown that it was reliable and dependable to work with.

At this point, I did not want to go back to either of the plastic surgeons I had talked to earlier. Quite frankly, I did not trust their judgment or motivation. I thought the first plastic surgeon was more concerned about trying to repair a poor job and maintain his reputation than he was in my well-being. The second seemed to be looking for patients on whom to try his new technique.

Grandstaff said she had seen some very good results by a plastic surgeon, Fred Tomlinson, who practiced in the Bay Area. I made an appointment that same week and could not have been happier with him. I told him there was some disagreement over whether anything could be done and, if so, what. I made it clear that I was there for information and did not want to pursue reconstruction if I did not have a reasonable chance of achieving attractive results. I also confessed that I was beginning to get paranoid around M.D.'s. I hadn't started out that way; I was learning it through experience.

"We have a lot to talk about," he said. During the rest of the hour—the time he allots to all new patients—he reviewed all my options for breast reconstruction and told me that even with my radiation and radical surgery he thought I should be able to get acceptable results. He shared Grandstaff's feeling that the muscle flap rotation would be the best procedure for me. He also showed me before-and-after pictures of women whose breasts had been reconstructed following both modified radical and radical mastectomies.

Where one plastic surgeon had seemed exasperated with my questions, and another had told me he "didn't like my attitude" (without elaborating on exactly what he didn't like) and had refused to show me pictures "because he could not promise the same results," Tomlinson seemed to enjoy answering questions and was pleased to show his work and tell me the number of breast reconstructions he had performed.

I took more time to check out his credentials. I found that he was one of the first plastic surgeons in the area to offer breast reconstruction. He had started as a surgeon, practiced for four years, then trained as a plastic surgeon and practiced for eleven years. Before entering private practice he had been head of plastic surgery at Letterman Military Hospital, a position in which he did a great deal of work on injured and mutilated soldiers returning from Viet Nam.

The surgeon I went to for routine checkups also investigated his credentials and abilities and agreed he would be a good choice and was someone who was very familiar with skin rotation procedures.

There was only one thing left to do—set the date for my operation.

The day before I entered the hospital, I thought seriously about canceling the surgery and enjoying a vacation instead. I pondered, "Where can I go with a suitcase full of books and hospital bed wear? No," I told myself, "you can't go through this again. It's time to get the experience behind you—whatever the outcome."

In my hospital room, my attitude began to change. There I talked to the plastic surgeon and the anesthesiologist and was visited by a surgical nurse who stopped in to review the procedure for the next day. I was beginning to feel relaxed and prepared for the surgery.

Surgery began around nine the following morning and continued until one in the afternoon. I remember waking and hearing Dr. Tomlinson say that all had gone well. This time I was surprised at how great I felt. Although my surgery had taken longer than I had anticipated, it was not considered a serious operation because it did not involve opening the chest cavity. As in all breast reconstruction, work was done at the superficial skin and muscle level.

I had some discomfort, but nothing that came close to pain. Four days after the operation, I was ready to leave the hospital, but first the bandages came off and I had a chance to look at the result. "I'm not going to look at it," I had said, at the same time eyeing my chest. I could not believe it. To my eyes, I looked beautiful. Sophia Loren could not compete.

Whereas before a large scar had run haphazardly, almost serpentlike, across my chest, I now had fine surgical lines outlining where the skin had been lifted and rotated to the chest area. I knew these scars would fade with time. The old skin was gone forever. I also was thrilled with the way the muscle filled in the washboard-appearing rib area where my chest muscles had been removed during my radical mastectomy.

I could have flown home. I think my enthusiasm stemmed not only from the fact that at last I had had a successful outcome, but also that my chest area looked so much better. Within three weeks I was back at work and jogging a slow mile. Within a month I was playing tennis. During the next six weeks, before the next steps—when the implant would be put under the skin and the nipple created—I found I had become somewhat of a novelty. But this time I was not going to object.

When I went to a surgical supply store to be fitted for a new arm sleeve (I occasionally wear one to control the swelling in my arm), a clerk asked if she could invite other clerks into my dressing room. "It looks beautiful," she said. "I've never seen anyone reconstructed following a radical mastectomy."

Later that week I was invited to the Stanford Medical Center for a "show and tell" program for some forty women who were considering reconstruction. It was part of Grandstaff's new program to give women accurate information on breast reconstruction. Several women were present who had had implants inserted following modified radical mastectomies as was one who had lost both breasts to cancer and had had them reconstructed. "How could doctors tell me reconstruction leaves a lot to be desired?" I thought. "These women look fantastic."

Now I come to the questions: Am I happier? Am I glad I did it? Has it been worth it? The answer to all three questions is a definite yes. Although the results are not perfect, there is no comparison between the before and after results. It seems strange and somewhat unexpected, but I feel more at peace with my body and myself. I don't blame my body for letting me down. I don't feel quite so victimized by a disease that not only threatened my life, but also deformed my body.

I look better when I face myself in the mirror. I enjoy not having to take part of me out of the drawer every day. I can wear the clothes that had to stay on hangers before and, more important, I have proved that you don't have to accept everything in life that you don't like.

Doomed to failure indeed!

*

It has been three years since my own reconstruction, and there are several details I want to add to complete the description of my experience. First, it took three additional outpatient operations before I was finished and achieved the best result I could expect. And although I was very pleased with the results of the first operation, it was not until the implant had been reduced and repositioned that I started thinking about it as a restored breast.

Many women will be interested in my husband's reaction to my surgery. Although it does not seem to have changed our relationship for better or for worse, he does appreciate the improvement. Perhaps he is only reacting to the additional pleasure I have received from looking better in my clothes or in being able to fill out a bra or negligee. But neither of us gives it much thought: My reconstructed breast is just another part of me, like an arm or a leg. I personally believe that the woman who decides to go through with this operation to please a man, rather than herself, is making a mistake.

I also believe that I paid a very small price for prolonging my life. Most women who lose a breast to rid themselves of cancer must feel the same way. The luckiest day of my life was when I discovered the growth in my breast, for it meant I could start treatment that has given me years to enjoy life. Yes, the surgery could have been better, but when I weigh it against not finding the cancer and losing my life, I still consider myself fortunate.

I know that since my mastectomy in 1972, pressure from informed women and progressive doctors has turned treatment around. Strangely, what I envy most is not that women today are being given less disfiguring treatments, but that they are so much more involved in their options. What bothered me most about my mastectomy was not the operation, but the fact that my options were not explained and I was so ill informed. There was no reason for me to go under anesthesia not knowing whether I would lose my breast. Some women may choose not to know, but to this day it is the most painful memory of my mastectomy experience.

Some women who are now considering breast reconstruction for themselves tell me they wish they could be as calm and as brave as I seem. I'll share my secret: It's easy when the surgery is behind you. I'm happy they didn't see me when I was going through the decision making. There was a time when just entering the doctor's office left me shaking. I was grateful that Fred Tomlinson was in another room when I entered his patient examination room. If he had seen me when I first came in, he might have noticed my knees wobbling or my hands shaking slightly. The experience showed me a side of myself that I didn't know existed—a very vulnerable side. I have always considered myself strong and independent. I still think I am, but I know now that I can also be quite frail. It is difficult to be strong when you have little control of circumstances and begin to feel you can't trust people. I think the whole experience gave me new insights into human nature and my own resources.

People have told me that I have an especially good reconstruction from a radical mastectomy, which I obviously owe to the skill of the plastic surgeon. But I also feel that I deserve some credit, for it probably would not have turned out so well if I hadn't wanted to take more responsibility for my body. I put time into finding a good plastic surgeon and checked his credentials. I talked to someone who had seen the results of his work and had feedback from his patients. I found someone who took time to explain the procedure to me, and I chose a person I could trust and with whom I could continue to work should I need more surgery. I knew there were still potential problems, but at least I felt that I had chosen a skilled professional who would do his best and take my needs seriously. What angered me so much about the surgeon to whom I went for checkups in California and about the surgeon who performed my original radical mastectomy in Wisconsin was that they thought it was their job to probe my motivations and judge my reasons. Their responsibility was to give me information so I could make an informed and intelligent decision. When I had my front tooth chipped and had to have it capped or when I decided to switch from glasses to contact lenses, nobody sat in judgment, telling me, "Women don't need it," as my first surgeon in Wisconsin had, or asking "if I were having problems," as my California surgeon did. The vast majority of mastectomy patients are mature, intelligent women, capable of making their own decisions for their own personal reasons. What they need is information, not judgment. Women who do trust and respect their doctors will certainly ask their opinions and recommendations and feel free to discuss their own motivation.

I learned through my reconstruction that once I found people who put my case in perspective and took time to discuss all my options, my trust in the medical community began to return. The sad part is that no reason exists for lack of communication and animosity between women and their physicians. Perhaps it stems from the surgeon's lack of time and overly crowded schedules. Could it be that they need power and would rather be authority figures than advisers? Perhaps the fault lies with the patient who is emotionally upset and does not know the right questions to ask. Whatever the source of the problems, I hope this book can help to build better lines of communication.

Much progress is being made in the treatment of breast cancer today, but too often women are the last to be informed about developments. I would not have written this book if information were easily available or if my experiences were an isolated case. In too many instances, barriers and lack of information are the norm instead of the exception.

The problem is worse because women report that breast cancer is their number-one health concern today, the disease they fear most. I personally believe that if they had more facts and information, they would have less cause for fear. If ever there has been good news to report about breast cancer, it is available today.

Chapter 2 explains that your chances of one day finding a lump are quite high, but that most of these disorders should not cause concern. With new options today, many women need not have a lump removed under anesthesia. Should you require a surgical biopsy, you do not have to sign a consent form giving the surgeon the right to remove your breast if the lump proves to be cancerous. A new two-step procedure gives you time to make plans, prepare yourself for the outcome, and explore treatment choices.

New information is available to help you discover whether you fall into a high-risk category for developing breast cancer; it is also possible to learn what you can do to decrease your odds of developing the disease. When breast cancer is found early, you have an 85 percent chance of surviving five years and close to a 75 percent chance of living ten years. And a new category of cancers, discovered very early and called minimal cancers, have 90 percent survival rates at 20 years. These are among the highest survival rates for cancer patients. Today, the National Cancer Institute and world health experts predict that within this decade new therapies, like the adjuvant chemotherapy discussed in Chapter 6, will improve survival rates and result in cures for many more women with breast cancer.

Many health specialists believe that women have delayed reporting suspicious lumps and examining themselves because they did not want to lose a breast if they found cancer. Relatively new options for radiation therapy and breast reconstruction can help women avoid deformity if cancer is indeed diagnosed.

I have packed this book with the kind of information I wish had been readily available when I was making my decisions. I wasn't looking for promises and reassurances, only accurate and objective information. This is why I have included photographs that show both good and less than perfect results from reconstruction and radiation therapy. To make a realistic choice, one must consider benefits along with risks.

A Woman's Choice isn't intended to usurp the importance of consulting with your doctor. Many women are fortunate in having found informed and sensitive physicians to work with. But, if you haven't, you should know that there are other ways of getting legitimate information, and other doctors you can consult.

We are truly living in a time of transition in the treatment of breast cancer, when two intelligent persons can look at the same information and draw different conclusions, depending on their values and perspectives. I do not pretend to offer you medical advice, but I have tried to present up-to-date options. It is to be hoped you will never develop breast cancer or even find that you have a breast lump. But, if you do, whatever your decisions about treatment, how fortunate we are to have today's choices.

CHAPTER 2

A Lump: What Does It Mean?

"I was twenty-four and a new mother when I first discovered a lump in my breast. My reactions ranged from denial (It's my imagination) to irrational terror (What will happen to my baby if I die?). When I finally visited the doctor, I trembled throughout his examination. A simple procedure revealed a harmless condition called fibroadenoma, but it was weeks before I got over my fear of cancer."

That's how Abby Avin Belson described her experience of discovering a breast lump in an article for *Women's Day* magazine in 1978. Her panic was not unusual. It's a common dilemma as, by even a conservative estimate, 50 percent of women at some time in their lives develop breast lumps, abnormalities, or thickenings large enough to be felt.

What many women, including Belson, are surprised to learn is how many of these problems are perfectly harmless. Shakespeare could have been describing finding a breast lump when he wrote "Fear is more pain than is the pain it fears." Between 75 and 80 percent of breast lumps are benign, a word defined in *Webster's New Collegiate Dictionary* as meaning "of a mild character," "of a gentle disposition"— in other words, not cancerous. The lumps often disappear on their own.

That's what happened to me about four years after my mastectomy, when I discovered a strange-feeling object just underneath my nipple. It was the first suspicious lump I had noticed since my mastectomy, and I was scared. My surgeon found it easily and suggested I come back in about a month to have it checked. In the interim I tried to ignore the lump in my breast. I couldn't bring myself to examine my breast until the night before my appointment. When I tried to find the lump, it wasn't there. I carefully examined my breast again. It seemed to have vanished.

I was still scheduled into the outpatient operating room for the following day and thought it best to keep the appointment if only to make certain that I wasn't imagining my good fortune. The next day, neither the nurse nor the surgeon could find it. I drove back to work feeling happy and relieved that I didn't have to have a biopsy. I also felt rather proud of myself for going through the process like a mature, calm, composed adult. I was mentally patting myself on the back for not being ridiculous and getting upset, as many women who find lumps do.

When I parked the car, however, and pulled the key out of the ignition, my hands wouldn't stop trembling. I thought I was going to cry. I had to sit there for a few minutes, digesting the fact that I didn't have a lump after all. I didn't have cancer. How wonderful. Some women are quite demonstrative about their worries and concerns. I tend to downplay them, thinking, "I'm not going to get upset until I have something to get upset about." But I'm beginning to understand that all I'm really doing is shifting my fears to a subconscious level. A lump is hard to ignore. Still, it does help to know that the odds are in your favor.

"The majority of lumps that are operated on turn out to be either fibrocystic disease or fibroadenomas, both harmless," says Henry Patrick Leis, Jr., professor of surgery at New York Medical College and one of the world's leading experts on breast disorders. Fibrocystic disease, by far the most common disorder, is actually a catchall or "wastebasket" term used to describe a range of breast problems. In routine physical examinations, over one third of women between twenty and forty-five years of age show symptoms. Some doctors say the symptoms are so common that fibrocystic disease should be included in the category of normal breast variation rather than disease. The problems usually vanish after menopause, unless you are taking hormones or using hormone creams.

Leis says he can group the disorders into three categories, although symptoms frequently overlap. The first stage, which occurs in the late teens and early twenties, shows up as a painful, tender swelling in the upper, outer areas of the breast. The swelling is usually more prominent in one breast, and the pain stops after a menstrual period.

The second stage occurs chiefly in the late twenties and throughout the thirties. Areas of thickening develop in both breasts and, on examination, Leis says, "It feels as though one is sliding the hand over a plate of green peas." Usually these cobblestone nodules have only two dimensions (height and width). If they do develop depth, however, they may be difficult to differentiate from cancerous lumps.

Stage three occurs in the late thirties and throughout the forties, sometimes continuing into the early fifties. Leis explains, "There is often a sudden, dull pain, a feeling of fullness, or a burning sensation along with the sudden appearance of a smooth and well-defined lump in either one or both of the breasts." These lumps can be moved, are often fairly tender, and feel "like a balloon filled with water." The cysts are often spherical and can range from microscopic to golf-ball size. The sudden accumulation of fluid just before a period increases the size of the lumps, but they are likely to deflate immediately after the period. Deeply embedded, or in clusters, they too can mimic cancer.

The second most common benign disorder is fibroadenoma. Unlike fibrocystic disease it is usually not painful and the lump does not vary in size with your menstrual cycle. It occurs in young women, most commonly between the ages of eighteen and twenty-five; the lump is described as firm, round, and movable. Experts say it "feels like a rubber handball," or "a marble under the skin of the breast." If you develop this kind of lump in one breast, there is a 14 to 25 percent chance that it will also appear in the other. Even breast specialists say such lumps often feel like cancer and must be removed to ascertain that they are in fact benign growths.

What causes all these disorders? "The answer is that we don't know," said Gertrude Case Buehring, a cancer researcher and associate professor in the School of Public Health at the University of California at Berkeley. "The popular belief used to be that estrogen hormones released by the ovaries during the menstrual cycle caused the growths. But the consensus now is that benign abnormalities are caused by a complicated interaction among several factors. Hormones are important, but probably more hormones are involved than estrogen. Family history also plays a large role and some speculate that the cycling process itself—the constant rise and fall of hormones in the breast—encourages the benign changes." Although researchers are still in the dark about what causes benign breast disease, they report interesting new findings in ways to reverse its development.

Vitamin E helps reduce symptoms and completely eliminates breast lumps for some women, according to Robert S. London, director of reproductive endocrinology at Baltimore's Sinai Hospital. He treated twenty-six women with 600 international units of vitamin E per day for eight weeks. Four women were unaffected, but ten women's breast lumps disappeared completely and twelve reported some beneficial response.

Another researcher reports that he has achieved very good results by advising women with severe breast disorders to give up foods, drinks, and drugs that contain caffeine. (See the table for a listing of these products.) He asks them to abstain totally from tea, coffee, cola, chocolate, and certain respiratory drugs and painkillers containing the chemical compounds called methylxanthines. In 90 percent of close to 300 women, breast cysts, at least partially, and in some cases completely, disappeared. The women remained free of the problem as long as they followed their diets.

The findings were reported by John Peter Minton of the Department of Surgery at Ohio State University College of Medicine. He

---

Products Containing Caffeine*

Beverages		Mountain Dew	49 mg	Triaminicin	30 mg
(hot, 5 oz. cup)		Royal Crown	36 mg	Vanquish	33 mg
Coffee	110 mg	Tab	45 mg		
(percolated)		*Over-the-Counter*		*Prescription Drugs*	
Coffee (drip)	150 mg	*Drugs*		(per pill or capsule)	
Coffee (instant)	66 mg	(per pill or capsule)		A.P.C.	32 mg
Tea	45 mg	Anacin	32 mg	(with codeine)	
(5 minute brew)		Appedrine	100 mg	Cafergot	100 mg
Cocoa	13 mg	Coryban-D	30 mg	Darvon	32 mg
		Dexatrim	200 mg	Emprazil	30 mg
Beverages		Excedrin	65 mg	Fiorinal	40 mg
(cold, 12 oz.)		Midol	32 mg	Migral	50 mg
Coke	42 mg	Nodoz	100 mg	Repan	40 mg
Pepsi	35 mg	Permathene-12	140 mg	Soma	32 mg
Pepsi Light	34 mg	Prolamine	140 mg	Synalgos	30 mg

*Reprinted from *Good Housekeeping,* August 1980.

explained that cysts and breast pain started to disappear as early as one week after young women altered their diets to exclude caffeine. It took about eight weeks before most women in his study noticed any changes; it took much longer for symptoms to disappear in older women. "One sixty-six-year-old professor who was used to drinking eight glasses of tea a day started to see changes at the end of eight weeks but had to stick to the diet for two years for complete results," he said. Most of Minton's patients have advanced fibrocystic disease. "I'm dealing with women who have lumps all the time, not just pre-menstrually. They can't wear a bra at all. They can't sleep on their stomachs."

When Minton first reported his findings, he was asked if decreasing caffeine or methylxanthines in the diet might influence the develop-ment of breast cancer. He replied that the treatment would certainly not reverse existing cancer, but said, "I tell women who have a family history of breast cancer to cut out methylxanthines completely. We won't know for twenty years whether this has any effect."

A new drug called danazol—a synthetic male sex hormone—has reportedly brought relief from pain and tenderness in women with moderate to severe forms of fibrocystic disease. Danazol's disadvantages, however, are its high cost—more than $100 for 100 pills at two drug-stores I checked—and its side effects, which include irregular or stopped menstrual cycles, weight gain, and acne. A few women experienced excess hair growth, deepening of the voice, and decreased breast size. Some women who have taken the highest daily dosages (400 mg) have also had liver dysfunction.

Ten million women take various forms of birth control pills today, and many researchers have tried to determine whether use of the drugs affects the incidence of benign breast disease. According to Jennifer L. Kelsey, an epidemiologist at the Yale University School of Medicine in New Haven, of ten studies started since the 1960s, all but one have shown that women who are on the Pill have less breast disease than those who are not. She said, "There seems to be an overall 20 percent de-crease of fibrocystic disease among women on the Pill. It generally takes two to four years to show up."

Women with fibrocystic disease often ask if they are more likely to get breast cancer. The answer is a qualified yes, with a summary of medical literature showing that if you have fibrocystic disease, you are more than twice as likely as the general population to develop breast cancer.

However, new studies are starting to show that only certain categories of benign breast disease predispose you to breast cancer. Michael D. Lagios, a staff pathologist at Children's Hospital in San Francisco, is one of several researchers in the country who are trying to zero in on the exact types of disease that increase risk. He explained, "There are fifteen to twenty different categories of benign breast disease and only a few are considered precancerous or most likely to place you at higher-than-average risk of developing breast cancer."

Knowledge of the structure of the breast helps in understanding which forms of lumps are precancerous. The breast contains three types of tissue. Fat accounts for most of the breast—the more fat, the softer the breast. Fat in the breast tends to increase with age. Elasticlike connective tissue, like the fibers in an orange or a grapefruit, holds everything together. Epithelial tissue builds the functioning part of the breasts, for example, the ducts and lobules, the branched network that runs from deep within each breast to the nipple. Think of the system as a tree that starts at the nipple and branches into ducts that get smaller and smaller until they end in the twiglike lobules. The only function of this elaborate system is to supply an infant with milk. Although many problems can develop in any of the tissues of the breast, 99 percent of disorders develop from the epithelial tissue, specifically the cells that line the milk ducts. Recent research suggests that the majority of benign, precancerous, and cancerous growths start to develop in the ends of the ducts—the lobules.

Only three types of benign breast disease that develop in these lobules are now believed to be "premalignant." That means if they develop in your breast, studies show that you have a threefold to fivefold increased chance of having a cancer someday develop in your breasts. In medical terms, the premalignant diseases are apocrine metaplasia, lobular hyperplasia, and ductal hyperplasia (also commonly called ductal papillomatosis).

But Lagios stresses that only the "atypical" forms of these disorders—the forms in which cells viewed under the microscope appear the most unusual and are grouped together in the most bizarre patterns—place you at higher than average risk. So, if your doctor tells you that you have the disorders without the atypical characteristics, your

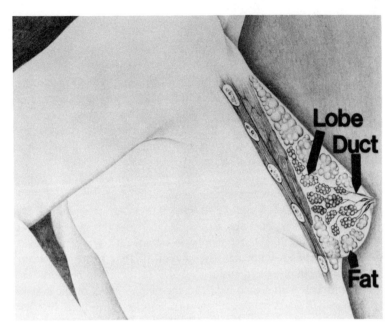

Arranged within each breast, like spokes on a wheel, are approximately 20 lobes. These lobes are subdivided into lobules and end in tiny milk producing bulbs called acini. The lobes, lobules and acini are connected to the nipple by a complex network of ducts that enlarge as they enter the nipple. (Picture courtesy National Cancer Institute.)

risk isn't any greater than that of other women in your age group.

Although these categories of benign disease are most likely to be associated with later breast cancer, there are some additional gray areas. For example, some noted researchers contend that women with gross cysts (larger than one-tenth inch in diameter) are more than four times as likely to develop breast cancer as women in the general population. Other highly regarded researchers have concluded from their studies that these cysts don't predispose women to breast cancer.

Lagios explains that although information on premalignant disease is evolving, most studies are based on only several hundred women and that exact interpretations may change. "The reason for increasing your

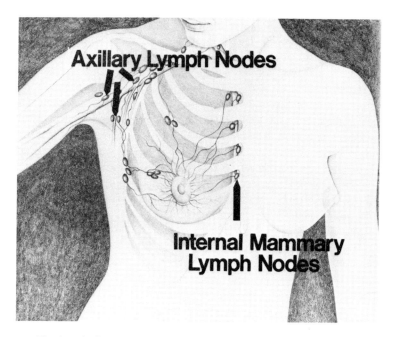

The lymphatic system removes wastes excreted from all body tissue and carries the fluid of the immune system throughout the body. Each breast contains a network of lymphatic vessels that drain either into the lymph nodes of the armpit or into the internal mammary lymph nodes. (Courtesy of the National Cancer Institute.)

knowledge," he said, "is that it helps you plan and live a little better. It also helps allay fears."

Certainly, there is reason for peace of mind if your biopsy report comes back showing that your suspicious lump was neither cancerous nor one of the benign diseases that increases your risk of getting cancer. But what about the woman whose breast lump falls in the possibly precancerous categories? Some physicians now recommend that she have a prophylactic mastectomy, which involves the removal and reconstruction of the breast.

But many physicians are more cautious. Pathologist Donald Earl

Henson of the National Cancer Institute's Breast Cancer Task Force said he would be more concerned if the abnormality showed up in a woman who had a personal or strong family history of breast cancer than if it occurred in a woman without a high-risk history.

Lagios also takes a cautious stand. "We know with some family histories, women have a 50 percent risk of getting breast cancer during their lifetimes. These women are simply carefully followed by their physicians so if cancer develops, it will be caught early. Then there are some physicians who say that we should remove a woman's breast on the basis of a pathology report that shows atypical growths that put a woman at fivefold increased risk—equivalent to a 45 percent lifetime risk of breast cancer. In some respects, medicine isn't consistent. It puts more emphasis on a pathological diagnosis than on a family history. That doesn't necessarily make sense."

The problem becomes even more frustrating because many pathologists don't give detailed reports on the benign breast lumps removed during a biopsy. They simply label them "fibrocystic disease." Many breast specialists complain about this practice, but women may have to insist upon more definitive answers themselves before changes are made. If you have a biopsy, you should make certain that your physician tells you exactly what type of abnormality the pathologist found, even if the pathologist must take a second reading to give you the information.

Another question that requires an answer is: How do these precancerous lesions become cancerous? Some contend that the benign tumors produce new cells that are cancerous. Others say that the benign growths don't actually produce cancer cells, but are only the result of the same conditions that cause cancer. The issue is far from settled.

Yet few dispute that when you do find a breast abnormality, you should not delay in making an appointment to have it checked out. It's true that most breast abnormalities are not cancerous, but it's also true that early treatment is your very best weapon against advanced spread of the disease.

It can sometimes be difficult to take responsibility for your health even when you're trying. A middle-aged woman told a nurse, "I don't know what I should be looking for. I have always had lumpy breasts. How do I know when I have a lump that I should be concerned about?"

It's a good question, but many women know intuitively when

something is wrong. That's why they almost always find the lumps themselves. The nurse's reply was excellent: "Even when you have lumpy breasts, you can find a hard lump. It's like finding a pea in a carton of cottage cheese."

The best advice is simply to look for a change of any kind. "One of the best ways to detect change is through routine breast self-examination," says San Francisco nurse Cathy Coleman, a specialist in breast cancer and breast care. "The goal is to get to know your breasts through regular, thorough, deliberate physical examination and visual inspection. The rationale is that it is easier to find a change from what is normal when you know what normal is."

Some experts believe that using soap or oil on the breast helps to feel differences more easily. Other cancer specialists suggest that every woman should get a thorough examination by an expert at least once in her life. That way, she'll have a better idea of what a good examination really consists of and can start to make a mental map of her personal contours and learn to recognize a change.

"Studies have shown," says Coleman, "that the woman who is most likely to practice breast self-examination is the woman who has received individual instruction from a health professional, particularly a physician. It takes about fifteen minutes a month for a thorough examination. Young women should do it a week after their period begins—the easiest time to spot changes—while women who are past menopause should pick the same day each month that they will remember."

Most pairs of breasts are symmetrical. If you find something that feels strange in one breast, check to see if you can find the same problem in the other breast. If you can, it's a good sign that you're not feeling cancer. Many a woman has become unnecessarily alarmed over a lump that was nothing more than a prominent rib.

Women shouldn't feel guilty about not practicing breast self-examination, Coleman says. Her message is that every time you give yourself an examination, you are giving yourself a bonus. It's also important to realize that it's not your job to find cancer, but only to note changes, and if you find a change, to seek prompt attention. "Women who give themselves breast self-examinations come to the clinic more often. We would rather have more women come in often with lumps that aren't cancerous than have the woman with a true cancer come in too late. It's finding the small tumors that makes us think we're making progress." She advises women who are too nervous to examine their breasts to have it done by a physician. And she encourages all women to ask for a breast examination during any regular medical examination.

Several months ago, I was working at home when the phone rang. It was Susan, a woman who teaches at the Berkeley campus. She's usually a most self-assured woman, but that day she sounded flustered. It took only fifteen seconds to find out why she had called. "I've got a lump," she said, "and I want to know what's going to happen."

"If you found a lump, the first thing you should do is to make an appointment to have it examined. Make the appointment today," I advised.

"My doctor was the one who found it," Susan said. "He wants to wait until after my menstrual period before he examines it again. I only thought of my questions after I left his office. I know I can either stick my head in the sand or try to find out as much as possible. Do you think I'm overreacting? Do you think it's stupid to ask these questions?"

"Susan, I don't think you're overreacting at all. It's better to know too much than too little. I think you're smart to investigate. Besides, what more valuable possession do you have than your own body and your own health?"

"I think it will just make me feel better," she said.

"O.K., I'm not a doctor, but I can tell you what doctors have written about how breast lumps are treated today. First, does your breast hurt?"

"Yes," she said, "it's really sore."

"That's a good sign. I know it's ironic, but cancer doesn't usually hurt. Fibrocystic disease, which is harmless, often does."

"Your doctor probably spent a good deal of time just feeling your lump and trying to move it. Right?"

"Right," she said.

"That's because you can get a fair idea if a lump is a harmless cyst or if it is a cancer by the way it feels."

I explained that, unlike harmless cysts, a cancer is often a single, hard, painless lump. It's found most often in the upper, outer section of the breast and, for unknown reasons, is more likely to occur in the left breast than in the right.

I told Susan that her doctor had tried to move her lump because benign growths are often easy to move, but a cancer is more likely to invade and fix itself to surrounding tissue, causing the breast to form scar tissue around the tumor. Other signs of cancer are hard irregular nodes under the armpit, skin dimpling, or a recent inversion or pulling in of the nipple.

Susan asked, "Why did he want me to wait?"

I thought he suspected that she had a benign cyst, which often disappears after a menstrual cycle. Cancer doesn't.

"What if it's still there when I go back? What will he do?"

I told her what I had learned at the 1981 Conference on Breast Cancer: If her lump had smooth borders characteristic of a cyst, a simple and reasonable choice of treatment would be fine needle aspiration. Using a syringe with a fine needle, her doctor would simply withdraw fluid from her tumor. For further information about the tumor's composition he would smear cells obtained from the biopsy on a slide for microscopic examination. If the fluid came out clear and the lump disappeared—and couldn't be felt in a follow-up examination a month or two later—chances were excellent that she had a cyst. And that would be the end of the treatment. She would not have to go into a hospital, would not need an anesthetic, and would not have a scar.

Susan's lump did not disappear with her menstrual period. Her doctor performed the needle aspiration, and the cyst deflated like a balloon rapidly losing air.

More and more doctors feel comfortable using this procedure to probe well-defined cysts, but they don't like to rely on the process to actually diagnose cancer. Studies have shown that this procedure may fail to detect the disease in 6 to 25 percent of cases. Doctors will continue the diagnosis if they doubt that the lump is just a cyst, find blood in the fluid, still feel a lump after all the fluid has been withdrawn, or find suspicious cells in the fluid sample.

Had Susan's lump felt like a mass of tissue rather than a cyst, her doctor could have performed a wide-needle biopsy. In this option, which would have required a local anesthetic, the doctor would have removed a thin core of tissue. Critics contend, however, that even this procedure doesn't provide a foolproof diagnosis. Benign and cancerous cells are often mixed together in a lump, and it is possible that the wide needle will remove only benign tissue, or, equally serious, miss the lump completely.

The most common reason a woman has a biopsy is that she has discovered a breast lump. Fluid coming from the nipple is the next most common signal that a biopsy is in order. While health specialists once believed that any fluid, except milk from a lactating woman, was a cause for concern, they now know that many normal and healthy women produce fluid in the ducts of their breasts, even when they aren't pregnant or breast-feeding.

Certain colors and consistencies of fluids create more suspicion than others. New York surgeon Leis is concerned when the discharge is pink, bloody, clear, or yellow, but not necessarily when it is milky, multicolored, or sticky, because such fluids aren't usually linked to cancer. If you are over fifty or the fluid comes from only one breast or a lump is present, you should definitely seek medical advice. But remember, most women with discharge are most likely to have benign disease. Leis found only 67 cancers in 503 women who came to him with spontaneous discharge. Another 96 had lumps that he considered either precancerous or highly likely to become precancerous.

There are numerous procedures for finding cancer as early as possible, even when no lump is present and for determining whether a lump is actually cancerous. With the exception of the surgical biopsy, they have one thing in common: They can't guarantee 100 percent accuracy. Each has its advantages and disadvantages. Some are more effective for younger women, others for older women. Some may fail to detect cancer in many cases, but pick up abnormalities the size of a pinpoint in others. The fact that all these tests exist and can be used in combination offers the best hope for early diagnosis.

Mammography, an x-ray of the soft tissue of the breast, is probably the least understood and most controversial diagnostic tool. It is also the most reliable technique for detecting cancerous tumors so small that they can't be spotted by physical examination. Two large studies have already shed considerable light on the benefits of mammography.

In 1963, the Health Insurance Plan of Greater New York offered free annual screening examinations with mammography and physical examination to a group of 31,000 women, who were compared to a similar-sized control group that received no unusual medical care. A nine-year follow-up study found the death rate from breast cancer had decreased by about 30 percent in the women fifty or older who had undergone mammography and physical examinations. So far, the survival rate of those who did get breast cancer has been best among the group whose tumors were detected with mammography alone. Another critical difference was that more than 70 percent of the cancers detected by mammography had not spread to the lymph nodes at the time of surgery. In contrast, only 46 percent of the women who found their lumps themselves had cancer-free nodes.

The success of the program led in 1973 to an even larger study in twenty-seven screening centers established by the American Cancer Society and the National Cancer Institute. The plan was to monitor some 280,000 women between the ages of thirty-five and seventy-four through physican examination, mammography, and thermography (a test that records the heat patterns of the breasts), for five consecutive years with five years of follow-up. Total cost of the study came close to 85 million dollars.

By 1977, 734 cancers had been detected. Mammography alone had picked up 45 percent of all the tumors. Most important, it was 95 percent effective in spotting small tumors (less than one half inch across) at a stage when 70 percent had not yet begun to spread to nearby lymph nodes.

Partway through the study, concerns over the possible long-term hazards of radiation to young women resulted in new guidelines, still in effect, which suggest that mammography be considered only for:

All women over fifty.

Women between forty and forty-nine who have had breast cancer or whose mothers or sisters have had breast cancer.

Women over thirty-five who have had breast cancer.

However, before the restrictions were imposed, approximately one third of the cancers detected in the centers were found in women under fifty. That's one reason the American Cancer Society and the American College of Radiology now suggest that all women have one mammogram taken when they are between thirty-five and forty years old. This pattern of the normal breast can be compared to future pictures, making it easier to detect early signs of trouble.

Ann Wallace, an active Reach to Recovery volunteer, feels that she owes her life to mammography. "It was luck. I was really in the right place at the right time. I had just turned thirty-six and was vice president of Merritt Hospital's volunteer auxiliary in Oakland when one of the twenty-seven breast-screening centers opened at the hospital. Hospital volunteers had a chance to go through the program before it was officially opened to the general public. I wasn't giving myself routine breast examinations. I didn't have a family history of breast cancer and I hadn't felt anything unusual in my breast, but I thought, 'Why not try it?' A few days later, I was informed by a letter that the mammogram had spotted something suspicious and that I should see a doctor. He ordered another mammogram and it was still there. The surgeon who examined me couldn't feel anything, even though he knew where to look."

"The tumor was under a third of an inch in diameter and was located very deep in her breast, close to her armpit," explained her Oakland physician, Calvin F. Lemon. "Even during the biopsy, the lump was difficult to detect and the surgeon had to remove the area where it had appeared on the mammogram. It turned out to be ductal carcinoma (the most common form of breast cancer that originates from cells that line the breast ducts) and one of twenty-one lymph nodes contained cancerous cells." Lemon estimates that it would have taken at least another several months before the lump would have been large enough to be felt by palpation, examination with the hands.

Ann's surgery, a modified radical mastectomy, took place eight years ago. Today she lives with her husband, Ken, in the Lake Tahoe area of California. She has had no recurrence of cancer and is the first to say, "If I hadn't had that mammogram, I probably wouldn't be here today." She adds that it was a fluke that she got the mammogram because new guidelines were soon to come out saying that screening should be limited to older women.

The benefits of mammography are known, but unfortunately, risks from the procedure still aren't completely understood. Formulas, based on what happens when women receive high levels of radiation, suggest that there really is no safe level. It is estimated that the radiation itself could cause between three and seven excess cases of breast cancer each year among a group of one million women who were screened with one rad of radiation from a single mammogram. It would take the cancers a minimum of ten years to develop.

But these theoretical statistics have to be balanced against the known yearly natural occurrence rate of breast cancer in one million women: 800 cases in forty-year-old women, 1,800 cases in fifty-year-old women, and 2,500 cases in sixty-five-year-old women. Mammography could help detect these cancers at an early and curable stage.

It's difficult to put the risks in perspective, but Stephen A. Feig, professor of radiology at Thomas Jefferson University Hospital in Philadelphia, tried during the 1981 Conference on Breast Cancer. "The low-dose risk from mammography is neither proven nor disproven," he said. "Studies show that the risk, if it exists, is very small and lowest to women over thirty years old." He said that today's levels of radiation in mammography carry the same risk as 400 miles of travel by air, 60 miles of travel by car, smoking three quarters of a cigarette, one and a half minutes of mountain climbing, and ten minutes of being a man over sixty.

Still, nobody can offer complete guarantees, and each woman must decide for herself if the immediate risk of having an undetected cancer outweighs her concern over the possible long-term risks from radiation.

Let me stress that no one disputes the necessity for a woman who has a suspicious lump or is at high risk of developing cancer to have a mammogram. The question under debate is whether women in the general population, who do not have symptoms, should have routine mammogram screening.

Unfortunately, no guidelines evolved from the special working group set up to review the encouraging findings from the twenty-seven national screening centers. Because participation in the screening had been voluntary, the review committee could not conclude that the women represented the true population. They wondered whether the group had included a disproportionate number of women who knew they were at high risk and so volunteered. Without a comparison group, they said there was no way to know for certain if cancers would have been diagnosed without screening and at what stage they would have been found. The working group called for a new randomized, controlled study to resolve the issue.

One doctor explained that, in his view, such a trial would be impossible today. "Not only would it be far too expensive, but with what we now know about mammography, we know in our hearts that the control group that didn't have the screening would have higher death rates from breast cancer."

However, one such study is already under way in two counties in Sweden. Some 90,000 randomly selected women over thirty-nine years of age who have no symptoms of breast cancer are being screened by mammography alone. Their breast cancer incidence and survival rates will be compared to thousands of their neighbors in the same counties who have not been invited to receive a free screening. Early results show that for every two cancers picked up in the women who are not receiving mammography, seven are being detected in the study group. So far, only 1 percent of cancers detected in the screened group had spread to the nearby lymph nodes.

Final results will carry considerable weight in determining the true value of mammography in screening the general population, especially for women under fifty. The study could also set new guidelines for how often women should have the test. Today's recommendation for an annual test is only an arbitrary suggestion. In Sweden, women between the ages of forty and fifty-five receive a mammogram every year and a half, because cancers grow especially fast in that age group. Women over fifty-five receive the test every two and a half years.

One word of encouragement is that the radiation dose of mammography is continuing to decrease from the 8 to 12 rads (radiation absorbed dose) given in the 1960s. One San Francisco breast clinic already has an instrument that gives clear, readable pictures by exposing the outer surface of the breast to doses under three tenths of a rad. The midsection of the breast (the place where most cancers develop) is exposed to still lower levels (only .02 rads). And when I went back to my community hospital, I found that the instrument they had been bragging about last year, which only exposed women to 1 rad of radiation, would soon be replaced by a new even lower-dose instrument. The switch to low-dose mammography is part of a national trend. By making a few phone calls, you may find a facility in your area with a low-dose instrument.

The American Cancer Society and the National Cancer Institute say that you should not receive more than 1 rad per examination. Several sources suggest you check the rad level with the radiologist or with your physician before you arrive for your appointment. If the dose is more than 1 rad, try to find another facility with lower-dose equipment. As a general rule, a teaching hospital or a large city medical center has the newest machines that expose women to the minimum x-rays for a good picture.

The decreasing radiation levels, combined with stories of women like Ann Wallace, are forcing some doctors to challenge the National Cancer Institute's guidelines of limiting mammography to women over fifty or only younger women at high risk. Radiologists state that mammography has an overall 85 percent success rate of finding cancers. It is least effective in taking pictures of the denser breasts of young women. One of its main advantages is that, unlike any other diagnostic tool, it can spot small microcalcifications—small bony deposits—which in Lagios' experience at Children's Hospital in San Francisco prove to be cancerous in one out of three cases biopsied.

In standard mammography, two pictures are taken of each breast, (but the newer instruments only take one view of each breast). At present, two processes are available, xeromammography and the older version, sometimes called film-screen mammography. "Today you can get good results from both with dosages under 1 rad. The question isn't which kind you should have, but how you can get a good test," explains Wende Logan, a radiologist and consultant to Roswell Park Memorial Institute in Rochester, New York. She advises: "Ask the radiologist which type is being used. If the answer is xeromammogram, it's O.K. If the answer is mammogram or film screen, ask if the breast will be compressed, a process that helps flatten your breast and leads to better results. If it is, then that's fine too. If it won't be squeezed, then go elsewhere." (The film-screen instrument that doesn't compress your breast was more than likely not designed to take pictures of your breast and the results often aren't as reliable.)

A San Francisco radiologist suggests that you try to find a facility in your area that has "dedicated" equipment—that is, equipment only used for mammography, because such equipment is more likely to produce better pictures. A facility whose staff cares enough to have dedicated equipment is more likely to have a good radiologist who is interested in quality diagnosis of breast problems.

One technique you're likely to hear more about is ultrasound, a process that relies on harmless sound waves—not radiation—to find abnormalities in the breast. The navy uses the technique to spot submarines, and sophisticated seafarers use it to find whales and large fish. Quite simply, high-frequency sound waves, when directed toward a particular site, return an echo pattern that varies with the kind of object they run into. Inside the breast, the sound waves will travel through a fluid-filled cyst, but bounce back from a hard tumor that could be cancerous.

The patterns are recorded as pictures on a televisionlike screen and videotaped for playback and later examination. Newer machines are programmed to penetrate the breast in a step-by-step fashion. The process is similar to examining an entire loaf of bread, one slice at a time.

The pictures are taken while you lie on your stomach on a comfortable table with your breasts immersed in a warm-water bath. This test may sound strange, but in my experience, it was relaxing and comfortable. I found out about ultrasound and tried the procedure at the San Francisco Breast Evaluation Center, which is under the direction of Philip B. Kivitz, a diagnostic radiologist who has worked with both ultrasound and mammography since 1966.

Kivitz, who finds it difficult to restrain his enthusiasm for the promising future for ultrasound, said the instrument, one of thirty in the country, takes an average of 250 pictures of each breast. Early machines, he said, could help differentiate only between large fluid-filled cysts and hard tumors. But the newer machines, he added, especially with their improved focusing powers, can detect abnormalities as small as one fifth of an inch across.

The hope is that, with more knowledge about the patterns, radiologists may one day be able to tell whether a hard tumor is benign or malignant. At this time, surgical biopsy is the only way to be certain. The limitations of ultrasound, he said, are that it is not as sensitive to the breasts of older women, which are composed mainly of fat, as to those of younger ones, and is not as good as mammography at spotting large bulky tumors or microscopic calcifications that may in fact be signs of cancer.

It is still too soon to recommend the procedure for routine screening of women who have no symptoms of cancer. "The main reason," said Kivitz, "is that we don't know how many cancers might be missed by the technique. That decision must rest on results of large-scale tests. The best estimates today are that for every hundred tumors, ultrasound will spot eighty-five abnormalities, but miss fifteen."

Although ultrasound needs extensive evaluation before it can be considered a replacement for mammography, Kivitz believes specific groups of women are most likely to benefit from the technique. They include those with dense breasts, those with fibrocystic disease, and those under thirty-five with breast problems. It could also be used for women over thirty-five who refuse x-ray mammography and as an alternative for pregnant women who have breast lumps.

You may also have a lump analyzed by a thermograph, an instrument that records on film emerging heat patterns from your breasts. The process stems from the knowledge that cancers usually produce more heat than normal tissue. To prepare for the test, you have to take off all your clothes above your waist and allow ten to fifteen minutes for your skin to cool. You will likely be asked to keep your arms away from your body, since even their slight contact against your breasts could make it more difficult for abnormal hot spots to show up on special heat-sensitive film. There is no discomfort associated with this test, except possibly from very tired arms and passing shivers.

The advantage of thermography is that it does not involve radiation. At this time, however, it is considered an experimental tool that has far too many disadvantages to be used for screening women who have no symptoms. Its accuracy varies widely, and some research reports that it detects only 40 percent of cancers. Also heat patterns may be affected by pregnancy and menstruation, and fat may insulate heat from being released from deep-seated tumors.

Although one study has indicated that a woman with an abnormal thermogram has a fifteenfold increased risk of developing breast cancer, the future role for thermography is still uncertain. Two things are clear, however: An abnormal thermogram is not justification for doing a biopsy and a normal pattern is not reliable enough to exclude women from further examination. (Interestingly, before my mastectomy, mammography—the process that has the best reputation for finding cancer—was unable to detect my tumor, probably because my breasts were firm and dense. Yet, thermography—the technique that doesn't have a good reputation for accuracy—spotted a problem that was interpreted to be "questionably positive" for cancer. The moral: No test is foolproof and each process has its stong and weak points.)

Some doctors use the Breast Pap Test (scientifically called Exfoliative Cytology of the Breast) to detect the earliest signs of cancer. The process involves analyzing breast fluid for abnormal or even cancerous cells. More than 60 percent of women produce fluid from at least one nipple if their breasts are gently massaged or a small suction cup is placed over a nipple.

Santa Barbara surgeon Otto Sartorius, who developed the suction device as a means of obtaining more fluid from the nipple, said the test is most successful for women between the ages of 40 and 60. So far, working with between 4,000 and 5,000 women he has diagnosed twenty-six breast cancers, eleven of which were smaller than a quarter of an inch in size and negative to both palpation and mammography. Sartorius believes that he has difficulty detecting a tumor larger than one third of an inch in diameter because by the time it grows that large, most tumors already have disrupted the ductal system that leads to the nipple, preventing the fluid from being easily expressed. Therefore, when this test is effective, it finds cancers at a small size when chances for cure and a good prognosis are excellent.

When he finds an abnormal cell in the fluid, he inserts a liquid contrast solution into the woman's ductal system through a hair-thin tube and takes an x-ray. Called contrast ductography, this process pinpoints the exact location of the problem. The next step is to remove the cells by biopsy. If the cells are cancerous, the woman can investigate options for treatment of early breast cancer.

Critics claim that the test is impractical because it detects so few cancers and because you often don't get fluids from both breasts. Sartorius believes that finding early cancer in even a few cases justifies the existence of the inexpensive and simple test.

Some women have complained that the Breast Pap Test causes discomfort. They say it feels as though their nipple were being pinched from the pressure of the suction cup. The discomfort most likely stems from the degree of suction, which can be controlled by the operator. I personally didn't find the test uncomfortable, but I fell into the group that didn't have any fluid.

A surgical biopsy, in which the lump, in whole or in part, is cut out from the breast, is the least convenient procedure for the patient, but offers close to 100 percent accuracy in telling the true character of a suspicious lump. The last few years have seen major changes in performing biopsies. The rule for decades in the United States was to perform all biopsies in the operating room with the patient totally asleep under anesthesia. If the breast lump proved to be cancerous, the policy was to continue immediately with a mastectomy.

Today, women have a choice between the one-step procedure and an increasingly popular two-step process, in which the doctor schedules the biopsy first and a mastectomy, or needed follow-up treatment, at a later date. In June of 1979 a panel of international experts were brought together by the National Institutes of Health to set national policy for the treatment of primary breast cancer. The panel recommended that a two-step procedure be done "in most cases."

Shirley Temple Black, who had a mastectomy in 1972, was the first woman I read of who opted for this procedure. She explained in a first-person story in *McCall's* magazine, "I find intellectually distasteful the prospect of waking up and finding that someone else had made a decision and taken an action in which I, lying quite inert on the operating table, had no voice . . . If my breast was going to be removed, I needed to be in on that decision. I wanted to take one step at a time."

Taking one step at a time makes sense for several reasons. If you know that you will have major surgery, instead of just a biopsy, you can make plans and arrangements for perhaps a week of hospitalization and several weeks of recuperation. You have time to consult a plastic surgeon, if you know that you want reconstruction, and to talk to a radiation therapist to find out if you would be a good candidate for breast-saving therapy with radiation treatments. The two-step process also costs substantially less than the one-step, which makes use of a fully equipped operating room for all patients. The most important advantage, however, is that it gives the pathologist time for a thorough and unhurried evaluation of your tumor. The information may justify a limited procedure in some cases, or it may indicate that you would do better with a mastectomy.

Surgeons once felt that a breast lump signaled an emergency situation. They had to act with all haste to remove the breast so the cancer cells would not have time to spread. In fact, it is now estimated that an average cancer has been present in a woman's breast for six to nine years before it can be felt. Delay of a few weeks makes little difference in prognosis and long-term survival, according to several studies.

The best cosmetic result from the biopsy scar comes when the surgical incision is made around the areola, the dark area surrounding the nipple, according to William W. Shingleton, a surgeon and director of the Comprehensive Cancer Center at Duke University Medical Center in Durham, North Carolina. "If that isn't possible, because of the location of the lump, an incision directly underneath the breast also gives good results." He explains that the subcuticular closing stitch, which runs under the incision, neatly bringing both sides of the skin together, results in the least obvious scar.

In either a one-step or a two-step procedure, it is critically important that an estrogen receptor assay (test) and a progesterone receptor assay be done if the excised tumor is cancerous. To be effective, the tests must be done immediately on the tumor tissue or the tissue must be frozen within fifteen minutes of its removal from the breast for later analysis. These tests help predict whether a tumor is dependent on hormones for growth, information that proves to be extremely

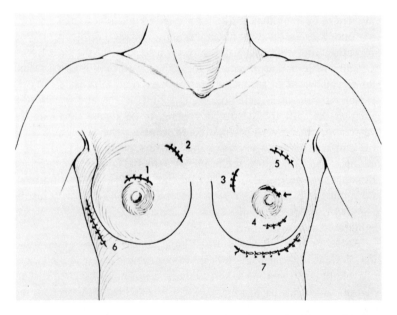

A breast biopsy doesn't have to result in a large noticeable scar. The best incisions result from following the natural wrinkle lines of the skin, which in the breast are circular around your nipple area (1 to 7). They very best cosmetic results come from incisions made around the areola (arrow) or under the natural fold of your breast. (From Cammarata, Angelo, et al., "Breast biopsy: surgical aspects, role of frozen section, and specimen radiography." In Gallager, H. Stephen, et al., eds, *The Breast*, St. Louis: C. V. Mosby Co., 1978.)

important should a cancer recur, even years later. For example, if a tumor thrives on estrogen, and if the tumor reappears at a later date, a doctor will know that he or she can induce a remission (the cancer will stop growing and possibly shrink) by treating the ovaries, because they are a key source for estrogen. Options include surgically removing the ovaries, irradiating them, or reducing the estrogen available to the new tumor with a newly developed antiestrogen drug (the current choice being Tamoxifen). However, a tumor that isn't estrogen dependent won't be affected by these treatments.

Researchers now know that about one third of tumors are strongly estrogen dependent, one third variably dependent, and one third not estrogen dependent. A June 1979 consensus conference called to discuss the value of the tests "strongly recommended that each primary tumor be assayed for estrogen receptor so that the assay information will be available when needed." The participants noted that the progesterone assay "adds appreciably" to information that helps predict how patients will respond to future therapy.

Both tests are fairly new, so you should find out before the biopsy operation whether the personnel and equipment to perform them are available at the facility in which your surgery will take place. However, if you have a very small tumor, there likely will not be enough tissue for both an adequate pathological diagnosis and receptor testing.

More good news about breast biopsies today is that it is usually possible to have the procedure while you are an outpatient. The operation can often be performed in the morning, and you are ready to leave in the afternoon. The two-step procedure is a boon for the increasing numbers of working women. They can return to work the next day, or sometimes the same day, with little discomfort.

Another improvement is that most breast lumps can be removed while you are under a local anesthetic, which leaves you free from pain but awake. Some instances when a general anesthetic is warranted are if a tumor is well over an inch in diameter, deeply embedded, or if the woman has other medical disorders. The woman's wishes are important—even if she prefers a one-step procedure. Some women prefer to go to sleep and trust the surgeon to do whatever is necessary. One woman told me that her biopsy was upsetting enough and she didn't think she was prepared to wake up and make all the decisions for a mastectomy. It is a personal decision based on the individual needs of the woman.

CHAPTER 3

Your Risk and What to Do About It

What is your risk of developing breast cancer?

Today, most women don't know. A 1980 National Cancer Institute report found that one out of every three women fears that she has a very real chance of getting breast cancer. In actuality, one out of every eleven American women—or 9 percent of the population—will develop breast cancer.

One person who isn't surprised that so many women have little realistic understanding of their risk is Patricia T. Kelly, director of a new genetic counseling program at Mount Zion Hospital and Medical Center in San Francisco. She is one of a handful of counselors in the country who have a program to help women evaluate their real risk. She said, "Many of the women I work with have grossly inaccurate beliefs about their own personal risk and the average woman's lifetime risk of developing breast cancer. One of my studies found that well over half of women (58 percent) substantially overestimate their risk, and close to one third of women (32 percent) greatly underestimate their chances of getting breast cancer. Only 10 percent had a realistic assessment of their risk level."

Before describing the factors that increase your chances of getting breast cancer, I want to stress what the odds really mean. They don't mean that you have a 9 percent chance of developing breast cancer during any one year. Rather, they mean that today's newborn baby girl has a 9 percent chance of developing breast cancer over her entire lifetime. Kelly says that what women often don't understand is that this lifetime risk figure is calculated on age up to 110 years old. The risk is considerably less during any one year. In fact, by the time you're sixty-five, you have only accumulated a three and one half percent chance of developing the disease. The percentage points add up much faster after menopause because older women are more likely to develop breast cancer than younger ones.

Surgeon Gordon F. Schwartz, in a paper he presented at the 1981 National Conference on Breast Cancer in San Diego, stressed that today's risk factors need to be put in better perspective. He explained, "If a woman reads a news story that says some factor doubles her risk of getting breast cancer, she immediately multiplies by two. The conclusion: she has an 18 percent chance of getting breast cancer. No wonder so many women are frightened."

He said that the 9 percent figure includes all women—those at the highest risk as well as those at the lowest. Schwartz said he would reduce the risk of the "normal" woman—the woman who doesn't have any of the major risk factors—to as low as 2 to 4 percent.

That leads into the second important point. Not all risk factors carry the same weight in forecasting whether you are likely to get breast cancer. The factors have to be divided into major and minor categories. The major factors are those that substantially increase your likelihood of breast cancer—age, a personal or family history of breast cancer, and some forms of benign breast disease. Doctors say that if you fall into these categories you should be examined more often than the general population.

There are literally dozens of minor risk factors, including when you started menstruating, when you had your first baby, whether you are white, Jewish, wealthy, overweight, where you live, and even if you have wet ear wax. Such factors can make you a little more susceptible to breast cancer than your next-door neighbor, but they aren't significant enough to make you follow an examination pattern different from your neighbor's.

The major risk factor for all women is age. The longer you live, the more likely you are to develop breast cancer, with 75 percent of all cases occurring in women over 40. The disease is extremely rare in children, and fewer than twenty-five well-documented cases have been reported in women under twenty. In Western countries, the incidence rate begins to climb after a woman reaches thirty. It increases rapidly as she enters her forties, levels off between forty-five and fifty-five, then continues its ascent, leaving postmenopausal women at highest risk.

The following chart documents the escalating effect of age, per 100,000 population: An estimated 25 women will have breast cancer when they are thirty years old, some 105 will have it when they are forty years old, and as many as 353 will develop it when they are eighty years old.

Family history can be a strong predictor of who gets breast cancer. It used to be believed that if your mother or a close relative had breast cancer, your chances of getting the disease were very high. Recent studies have shown that not everyone with a family history carries an especially high risk. The ages at which your relatives developed breast cancer and whether it involved one breast or two breasts are the crucial factors that determine your risk.

Patricia Kelly counsels women that they have a 50 percent chance of developing breast cancer during their lifetime if two close relatives—a

Average Annual Incidence Rates of Breast Cancer
Based on Census Data from 1973 to 1977

"Incidence in the U.S."

Age	White Women (per 100,000)	Black Women (per 100,000)
15–19	0.2	—
20–24	1	2
25–29	8	10
30–34	25	38
35–39	55	65
40–44	105	101
45–49	176	141
50–54	196	161
55–59	230	193
60–64	252	211
65–69	286	209
70–74	304	262
75–79	343	288
80–84	353	244
85 and over	376	261

Journal of the National Cancer Institute, Monograph No. 57, June 1981.

mother and a sister, for example—had cancer in both breasts when they were young (before menopause). But if those same two relatives developed the cancer in only one breast, and developed it after menopause, their lifetime risk drops to 16 percent. Similarly, if they have two sisters and each one had both breasts removed as a result of breast cancer before her menopause years, those women would run a 50 percent lifetime risk of breast cancer; that risk would drop to close to the national average if the cancers in their sisters affected one breast only and came after menopause.

In spite of the high risk associated with a strong family history of breast cancer, only 10 to 15 percent of women who get breast cancer have any family history of the disease. Stated another way, 85 percent of women who develop breast cancer do not have a family history of the disease.

Kelly explained that "daughters of women who had breast cancer are especially likely to overestimate their own risk. Many times daughters have been told by their doctors that they were at 'high risk' and interpreted that to mean that their chances were 80, 90, and even 100 percent of getting breast cancer. Sometimes these women were so frightened about getting breast cancer that they didn't give themselves routine breast self-examinations for fear of what they might find." Kelly added that other women whose mothers had breast cancer had told her they were thinking seriously about having their breasts removed as a safeguard against developing breast cancer themselves.

Thirty-one-year-old Ellen (not her real name) was one such person. Ellen had been urged by several physicians to have both her breasts removed and to have implants inserted, solely as a preventive measure. The advice stemmed from the ominous-appearing fact that her mother and three maternal aunts had all had breast cancer, each having had one breast removed after she passed menopause.

Kelly said, "Ellen had been told that her chances of getting breast cancer were 'very high' or 'close to 100 percent.' Yet, a more critical analysis of her family history with the new counseling information showed that her personal risk was no different from the national average. Had her physicians been aware of this risk information, it's unlikely they would have recommended that she have mastectomies."

Although it was commonly believed in the past that you could develop breast cancer only if it appeared in your mother's family history, genetic counselors now say that breast cancer risk can be just as readily transmitted through your father's side of the family.

A personal history is another major risk factor. It's well accepted that if you have had cancer in one breast, you have an increased chance of developing it in your second breast. Some people contend that your chance of getting cancer in your remaining breast increases by 1 percent each year after your mastectomy. Others say the risk increases by one fifth of that amount each year. So, at the end of ten years, if you have already lost one breast to cancer, you have a 2 to 10 percent increased chance of developing cancer in your second breast, depending on whose statistics you follow.

Studies show that if you have had a biopsy for benign breast disease, you have three times the normal risk for eventually developing breast cancer. This curious association probably stems from the fact that certain types of benign disease increase your odds of getting breast cancer three to five times over women who do not have the abnormalities. The fact that one lump has been removed does not mean that others with the same cancerous potential aren't left in the breast or that others won't develop in later years. A biopsy in itself doesn't place you in a high-risk group, but if the biopsy shows one of the precancerous tumors already discussed, doctors say you should be followed more closely than the average woman.

It would be hard for any woman not to have at least one minor risk factor. Such factors are so common and so diverse that many women probably have several. At this time, they are only items of interest compiled by epidemiologists—researchers who spend their lives tracking down all the factors associated with a certain disease, hoping that some may eventually give good clues to how and why problems develop. Until the true cause is understood, many of the factors will remain curious pieces of a complicated jigsaw puzzle. One epidemiologist joked that you could probably find an association between the number of television sets a woman owned and her risk of developing breast cancer: Breast cancer tends to strike women in higher socioeconomic groups; they own more television sets. The moral is that even a clear association can be difficult to interpret. The factors often don't have an obvious cause-and-effect relationship.

As an example, the first risk factor was noted as early as 1700 when an Italian physician, Bernardino Ramazzini, was investigating diseases of workers and noticed that nuns had an excess incidence of breast cancer. He guessed correctly that this wasn't caused by their occupational activities, but by the fact that they weren't married. Since that time, numerous studies from different countries have agreed that single women do indeed have higher rates of breast cancer. After those for single women, rates drop progressively for widowed, married, divorced, and separated women. Why women separated from their husbands have the lowest rates is as much a puzzle as why single women have the highest rates.

Several of the risk factors are related to your reproductive system, perhaps influenced by your body's hormone levels. These factors include the age at which you started menstruating and the total number of years of menstruation, when you had your first baby, when you entered menopause, and whether menopause was natural or the result of surgery. Girls who start menstruating at or before the age of 12 tend to have an increased risk of breast cancer. At the other end of the spectrum, women who enter menopause late in life, after 50 years of age, also have an increased risk. Risk is higher still when menopause occurs after 55. Although the increased risks are relatively small, the findings are interesting because during the last half of this century the beginning average age of menstruation has decreased from 14 to 12.5 years, and the average of menopause has increased from 47 to 50 years.

Some studies suggest that breast cancer patients have longer lifetime menstrual activity than women who don't get breast cancer. And the better nutrition among today's children is sometimes used to explain why girls mature faster and start their menses at earlier ages than their mothers and grandmothers did.

If you have had your ovaries removed, you have a 40 percent reduced risk of developing breast cancer. The protection is strongest among women who have them removed when they are under thirty-five. Older women still benefit, but the protection definitely decreases if you have the surgery when you are older. Finally, there are conflicting reports on whether women with irregular periods have a higher risk of getting breast cancer than women with normal periods.

It is now accepted that having a baby at a young age can reduce your risk of developing breast cancer. A 1970 international study looked at birth rates in seven countries in which the incidence of breast cancer varied from high to low. The findings were summarized in the January 1973 *Journal of the National Cancer Institute*:

1. Breast cancer risk increases with the increase in age at which a woman bears her first child. Women who have their first child before the age of 18 have about one third the breast cancer risk of those whose first delivery is delayed until age thirty-five or older.

2. To be protective, pregnancy must occur before age thirty.

3. The protective effect is essentially limited to the firstborn child. Subsequent births, even to a young woman, add little or no additional protection.

4. Protection is gained only by a full-term pregnancy. Abortion tends to be linked to an increased, not decreased, risk.

5. The protection gained by the early first birth lowers a woman's lifetime risk of getting breast cancer. It is still "in force" among women seventy-five and older.

The evidence suggests that the first pregnancy in a young woman has a "trigger" effect, which either produces a permanent change in the factors responsible for the high risk or changes the breast tissue and makes it less susceptible to cancer in the future. Some believe that the teenage years may be a critical period when breast cancer is actually initiated, but that it takes many years to develop. One theory holds that protection against the future development of breast cancer comes from the changed estrogen patterns that show up after the sixth month of pregnancy.

Interestingly, the woman who becomes pregnant after the age of thirty is four times more likely to develop breast cancer as women the same age who remain childless. The explanation is that older women are more likely to have small existing cancers, which may be stimulated by the rich supply of hormones released during pregnancy.

Most other risk factors are related to environmental influences, which range from your exposure to radiation to where you live and the food you eat. Exposure to high levels of radiation is linked to higher-than-average rates of breast cancer, as well as higher rates of leukemia and cancer of the bone, skin, thyroid, and rectum. Excess incidence of breast cancer has been found in atom bomb survivors, in women who received radiotherapy for benign breast disease, in women who received multiple x-rays for treatment of tuberculosis, and in women who received radiation for inflammation of their breasts after pregnancy.

Women with tuberculosis who were x-rayed an average of 102 times over several years showed an 80 percent increase in breast cancer, and the Japanese bomb survivors exposed to 90 rads (radiation absorbed dose) had two to four times the number of breast cancers found in women who hadn't been near the bombed areas.

Studies tend to agree that the breasts of older women are less susceptible to radiation than those of younger women. A critical time for exposure to radiation occurs in girls, between the ages of 10 and 19, when their breasts are undergoing rapid change and development. In fact, one study has found that no excess breast cancer appeared in Japanese women who were over twenty years of age at the time of the bombing and who were exposed to dosages under 100 rads.

The risk from low doses of radiation—as for the level used in mammography—is still debatable. If the risk exists, it is small and has never been observed.

The country, the state, even the county you live in is related to your risk of getting breast cancer, explained Nicholas Petrakis, chairman of the Department of Epidemiology and International Health at the University of California at San Francisco. He handed me a graph of different counties in the San Francisco Bay Area showing that rates can vary tremendously even in a radius of less than 100 miles. In Marin County, the wealthiest area, close to 100 women per 100,000 get breast cancer. In neighboring San Francisco County and in Alameda County, where I live, the rates are less than 80 women per 100,000. A National Cancer Institute monograph showed that the incidence varied from year to year, but still fit into a consistent pattern. With the exception of one year between 1969 and 1975, Marin County led San Francisco and Alameda counties in breast cancer by as many as 34 additional cases for every 100,000 women.

No one knows why women in Marin have such a high rate of breast cancer, but one woman who lived there asked a cancer researcher the obvious question, "Do you think I should move?" The cancer specialist replied, "Moving won't help. Remember that just as people select the area they live in, an area can select the characteristics and backgrounds of people who are able to live there."

Women who can afford to live in Marin County fall into a higher-than-average socioeconomic bracket, which has an increased risk of breast cancer. They probably also delay having children until they are older, which doesn't help their risk and, some believe, the eating habits they established early in life may affect their rate of incidence. The point is that those women certainly had a specific risk pattern when they moved into the area and will carry that high-risk susceptibility with them no matter where they live. Moving won't help decrease the odds of getting the disease any more than it would help to give up extra television sets.

Whatever the reason, women with relatively high rates of breast cancer live in the United States, Canada, Western Europe, New Zealand, and South Africa. Certain urban areas in the United States—San Francisco, Oakland, Minneapolis, St. Paul, Detroit, Pittsburgh—and the states of Iowa and Colorado in particular carry the highest risk. Small towns and rural areas provide the lowest risk. Intermediate rates occur in eastern and southern Europe, and rates of breast cancer are lowest in Asia, Latin America, and Africa. As an example, an average of 85 per 100,000 women develop breast cancer in the United States in contrast to 13 per 100,000 women in Japan.

The risk could easily be explained by genetic background if it weren't for the fact that, as women in countries with low breast cancer rates migrate to the United States, their rates climb above those of their country of birth. As Japanese women migrate to Hawaii and the continental United States, their risk increases from 13 to 47 cases per 100,000 women. The increase suggests that environment plays an important role, as perhaps do diet and earlier maturation and menstruation. The United States also has seen a rapid increase in breast cancer among black women. Some speculate that this could be linked to their moving into higher socioeconomic classes or changing their diet to conform to the average white woman's.

Only health food faddists used to contend that a change in diet could keep you healthy. But, geneticist Patricia Kelly says, "In the last few years, medical and scientific journals have published an increasing number of articles on nutrition and disease. I think the interest in nutrition will continue to grow and will lead to new ways of dealing with disease." She cautions that a lot of the information is still not definitive, but adds, "One point that seems to show up again and again is the high correlation between fat consumption and increased rates of breast cancer and colon cancer."

A study of fat consumption in 39 countries found that death rates from breast cancer were five to ten times higher in countries with high fat intake, with animal fats contributing more than vegetable fats to increased risks. Also, laboratory mice and rats fed high-fat diets show higher rates of mammary gland cancer than animals on low-fat diets.

Kelly points out that the breast cancer rate is especially low in Japan, where only 20 percent of the average diet comes from fat. In contrast, the breast cancer risk is high in the United States, where 40 percent of an average woman's calories come from fat. "An exception to this trend is in Finland, where women consume a lot of fat, but have a low incidence of breast and colon cancers. One explanation is that they eat a large amount of fiber, which might be protective in some way."

Studies with animals show that vitamins A, B, and C also decrease mammary gland cancer, said Kelly. Interestingly, the trace element selenium, commonly found in soil, may affect breast cancer risk. Small amounts of selenium are necessary in the diets of both humans and animals, and some recent studies, said Kelly, have suggested that the element might help protect against breast and other cancers.

A study published in the *Journal of Surgical Oncology* found that breast cancer patients had lower levels of selenium in their blood samples than the general population. Areas with low selenium levels in their soil also tend to have higher rates of cancer. Cities and locations with higher concentrations of the element in the soil have lower cancer rates.

However, excessive amounts of selenium are linked to problems in animals. Rats fed ten times more selenium than needed had increased rates of tumors, and animals who have grazed on selenium-rich soils have developed symptoms of "alkali disease" or "blind staggers." They became stiff, lame, lost their hair and sight, eventually became paralyzed, and died.

Several studies suggest that overweight, especially in the post-menopausal years, increases the risk of getting breast cancer. Theories suggest that fatty tissue stores cancer-causing agents from food and releases them into the bloodstream. Fatty tissues are also a rich source of estrogen. So the fatter a woman is, the more estrogen circulates in her bloodstream. It's now known that estrogen—at least in some women—helps tumors to grow.

Many women wonder if taking a birth control pill increases their risk of developing breast cancer. Most studies show there is no evidence that it does increase the risk. But the same studies unanimously agree that it is still too soon to draw definitive conclusions. The Pill has been available since 1962, and some researchers say that if it did result in an increased risk we would be in the middle of a cancer epidemic by now. The 1980 Multi-Disciplinary Project of Breast Cancer, however, reported that "the women who have been exposed to oral contraceptives are only now reaching the age of maximal risk to breast cancer."

One recent study, reported at the 1981 National Conference on Breast Cancer, did find that one very unusual group of women who had been on the Pill did have a higher risk of breast cancer. "We looked at a group of 170 women from the Los Angeles area who had all had breast cancer before they were thirty-two," said Brian E. Henderson, professor and chairman of the Department of Family and Preventive Medicine at the University of Southern California School of Medicine. His study reported that their risk of getting breast cancer was roughly doubled if they used the Pill for four years before having their first child. It was more than tripled if they took birth control pills for 8 years or more before their first pregnancy. The risk of getting breast cancer in the group was highest among the young women who also had a history of benign breast disease or who developed the problem after they started taking the contraceptive.

What was their conclusion? Does the Pill cause cancer—at least in some groups of women? Henderson said it is far too early to draw conclusions and certainly too soon to suggest that women get off the Pill on the basis of his one study. "I don't think that the findings belong in the general press," he said, "until researchers and scientists have had time to look at the information and interpret its significance."

Others will obviously try to repeat his study, but if the information is available to the scientific community, I think it should be reported to women who are taking the Pill. However, one study only presents a suggestion or a theory. Conclusions must wait until others observe the same pattern in their research with other women.

Another often quoted study has found that the Pill may accelerate the growth of a small preexisting cancer. California researchers Elfriede Fasal and Ralph S. Paffenbarger followed 1,770 San Francisco Bay Area women who had been on the Pill. Although these women did not have an overall higher incidence of breast cancer, two puzzling patterns emerged: (1) breast cancer was twice as likely to show up among women who had been on the Pill for two to four years, and (2) it was six to eleven times more likely to occur among women who had had a prior biopsy for a benign breast disease and who had been taking the Pill for longer than six years.

Fasal and Paffenbarger theorized that the Pill had accelerated the growth rate of small preexisting tumors, and that the cancers reached detectable stages after two to four years. "Doesn't this mean that the Pill can be hazardous?" I asked San Francisco oncologist (cancer specialist) Richard Cohen. "No, it only means that we're going to pick it up earlier than if the woman had not been taking the Pill. I don't think it calls for limiting the use of the Pill, but possibly for monitoring women more closely after they have been on the Pill for two years," he said.

The researchers explained, "The excess risk of breast cancer among women with a history of breast biopsies suggests that some have a potential for cancer that is activated by long-sustained oral contraceptive use." In this case, they say it's practical to recommend that women with a history of benign breast disease use another form of birth control.

The Food and Drug Administration estimates that three million women take estrogens for menopausal and postmenopausal symptoms. Are these women at higher risk of developing breast cancer? Estrogens have been administered for more than forty years now, and most studies show no association between use and increased risk of breast cancer. However, delayed risk was suggested by one long-term study of 1,891 women. Twice the expected risk of breast cancer showed up after fifteen years. Risk was highest among women who used higher-dosage tablets and developed benign breast disease after having started taking the drugs. Although the increased incidence rates could have been explained by other factors, the Multi-Disciplinary Project on Breast Cancer concludes: "Prolonged use of these agents, especially at high doses, should be avoided and . . . the possible advantages should be evaluated in light of a possible increase in the risk of breast cancer."

A highly controversial theory suggests that women at high risk for breast cancer have distinctive density patterns on their mammograms. Radiologist John N. Wolfe of Detroit has put the images into four groups. He contends that women with dense, glandular breasts (labeled P2 and DY) are more prone to breast cancer than women with less dense, fatty breasts (called N1 and P1).

Opponents have challenged Wolfe's findings, saying that breast patterns change with age and do not really identify the women who run a high risk for cancer. They also cite at least seventy-two different patterns and call the four-pattern scheme "simplistic." Those who disagree with Wolfe's theory claim that an increasing number of surgeons perform unnecessary prophylactic mastectomies based on the so-called Wolfe patterns. A National Cancer Institute follow-up study of some 40,000 women will help settle the debate, but until final results are in women should be cautious about having their breasts removed just because they fit into this highly debated high-risk group.

In addition to these frequently listed minor risk factors, there are numerous others. For example, women who have had cancers of the ovary, salivary glands, colon and some kinds of uterine cancer are at increased risk for developing breast cancer. The highest risk is for those who have had endometrial cancer—a malignancy of the lining of the uterus. This group develops 30 percent more breast cancers than expected. Risk is elevated for Jewish women—nobody knows why. Women who have a wet and sticky kind of ear wax also are at higher risk. This factor sounds absurd until you realize that ear glands and breast glands share certain physiological and anatomical characteristics. The same genetic traits that determine whether a person will have wet or dry ear wax could be closely associated with the trait that determines a natural tendency to get breast cancer.

Some researchers have tried to link stress and specific personality types to women who develop breast cancer. For example, the disease has been linked to loss or separation from loved ones, bereavement, an unhappy home life, inability to deal with anger, aggression, unresolved parent-child tensions, sexual disturbances, excessive childhood responsibilities, and excessive death rates of brothers and sisters. Others contend that the breast cancer patient has a tendency to withhold anger, hostility, and other negative emotions and, in essence, is "too good to be true."

So far, no consistent relationship has been found between stress and personality types and breast cancer. Some critics speculate that conditions like depression and anxiety are the result of the disease rather than a contributing cause. They also point out that personal losses, social traumas, and inability to express emotions characterize many persons, including those who never get breast cancer.

I personally dread reading these personality studies. They make me feel like a bug being thoroughly dissected, cell by cell, under a microscope. Isn't there any privacy? Sometimes I wonder why I couldn't have developed some rare disease that nobody had heard of instead of one that is so common and constantly in the news. Now I even have to wonder about my personality—whether I'm too pleasant or too nice. The only fortunate flipside is that when I do get angry at somebody or have a disagreement, I think it might at least be helping me combat a recurrence of cancer.

Many women believe than an injury to their breast increases the risk of cancer and that breast-feeding protects them against the disease. Both beliefs are old wives' tales, and the current scientific consensus is that neither is true.

Nicholas Petrakis explained that the only reason for studying all these risks is to attempt to identify variables in a woman's environment that might be manipulated to decrease her risk of developing breast cancer. He admits that in the case of breast cancer, very few factors can be controlled. "You can't tell women to become poorer because there is a positive correlation of breast cancer with high income. You can't go around telling them to have their first child before the age of eighteen because that is likely to protect them. You're running against the current social trends of delayed marriage and delayed pregnancy. Some studies show that risk factors aren't all that effective at predicting who actually gets breast cancer. There is a lot more to breast cancer than the risk factors we now know about."

It's easy to forget that risk factors are most effective at showing which groups of women are most likely to get breast cancer. When you apply that information to individuals, prediction is more problematic.

In my case, some risk factors were obvious, but I doubt that any red flag signaling high risk of breast cancer would have gone up if I had entered a doctor's office. I had started menstruating when I was 11, ahead of most other girls in my grade school. I was single and hadn't had a child by age twenty-five, but that wasn't supposed to work against me for years yet. As a result of a positive tuberculosis test, I had received as many as three chest x-rays when I was going through my teen years. Doctors I have asked say the dose was too small to initiate a cancer, an answer I'm not certain I agree with, especially since I received the radiation at an age when breasts are known to be most sensitive to radiation. I had been on birth control pills for nine months, something I suspect at least accelerated the growth of my cancer.

As regards family history, an important risk factor, my more than 60-year-old mother and my sister were and still are cancer free. However, I had a great-aunt who had had breast cancer, and one of my mother's four sisters had undergone two mastectomies before she entered menopause. Detailed information on the importance of family history for predicting risk still hadn't been reported in medical journals. But Patricia Kelly said if the material had been available and if I had come to her for risk counseling (before I had actually developed the disease), she would have estimated my lifetime risk to be between 11 and 25 percent. She added, "And I would have told you that it was most likely that your odds were closer to the lower estimate, which is only a little higher than the national average." Unfortunately, my tumor never got the message.

Surgeon Henry Patrick Leis, Jr., once described the "ideal" high-risk patient. He says in one of his many publications on breast cancer:

> The ultimate search for the woman with the highest risk of developing breast cancer would culminate in the finding of a 58-year-old obese, hypertensive, diabetic, white, Jewish convert nun with hyperthyroidism, receiving reserpine [chemical] therapy for hypertension and estrogens for severe climacteric symptoms; who is living in a cold climate in the Western Hemisphere; whose mother and sister had bilateral, premenopausal breast cancers, who has a wet-type earwax, a low estriol titer [measurement of natural estrogen level] and subnormal androgen excretion levels; who had previous endometrial cancer and cancer in one breast; who nursed from her mother, who had B-viral particles in her milk; whose menarche [beginning of menstruation] was at the age of 9; whose remaining breast revealed precancerous mastopathy on random biopsy, a DY parenchymal [Wolfe] pattern on x-ray examination, and abnormal thermographic findings; who is immunodeficient, with decreased T-lymphocytes; who received multiple fluoroscopies [x-rays] for tuberculosis therapy; and who lives on a diet high in fats.

Even if Leis could find his dream candidate, she could still surprise him by not having breast cancer. Despite this somewhat pessimistic perspective, there still are actions that women, especially prudent high-risk women, might consider. Petrakis, Leis, and Kelly are among the first health specialists in the country to make suggestions that could have a bearing on a woman's potential for breast cancer.

For starters, Petrakis suggests keeping one's weight down. He also cautions against unnecessary x-rays, especially ones of the chest for adolescent girls, whose developing breasts seem to be especially vulnerable to radiation. Since some studies show that added estrogens after menopause are a risk factor and others that they aren't, his advice is to get by with minimal use.

He also suggests that when physicians find breast cancer in a mother, they examine the whole family and relay risk information to the daughters. Finally, counseling for relatives of women with a known family history of breast cancer might lead to early diagnosis and treatment of incipient breast cancer.

Genetic counselor Patricia Kelly outlines dietary information for her patients who fall into high-risk groups, but again stresses that it is only speculation that diet will reduce their risk. "But we do know that decreasing the fats in the typical American diet won't hurt you, so why not try it?" she asks. Since studies suggest that people who eat less fat and more fiber have less breast cancer, she advises cutting down on meat, butter, and margarine and switching to low-fat dairy products.

She tells women about an article in *Preventive Medicine*, which suggests they eat more whole grains and cereals, more potatoes, rice and beans, and fresh fruit and vegetables. "I often show them a fiber cookbook and a French low-fat cookbook as two sources of menus," she says.

In addition, Kelly tells patients that selenium seems to make a difference. Grains, tuna, mushrooms, garlic, liver, eggs, and brewer's yeast are good sources for selenium. And she tells them that studies suggest there could be benefits from vitamins A, B, C, and E.

Leis thinks it is sensible for women to take a daily vitamin B complex and at least 1,000 to 2,000 mg a day of vitamin C. Although it is still not unequivocally established, some believe that vitamin C makes normal tissue stronger and reinforces the immune mechanism of the body against cancer. He advises taking the vitamin B supplement because the liver, which has to break down and detoxify many food products that may contain cancer-causing agents, functions more efficiently with the help of the vitamin.

He also recommends that women with a family history of breast cancer avoid the use of oral contraceptives.

Increasingly, women today are choosing a prophylactic mastectomy as a means of decreasing their chances of developing breast cancer. These women generally fall into one of two categories—they have either an above-average risk of developing breast cancer or an above-average fear of the disease. Many make the choice after having gone through the anxiety of repeated biopsies for lumps that proved harmless, but nonetheless left them wondering if they did have cancer. Although the option has been available for decades, it has only recently begun to gain popularity, possibly because it can be done more successfully today. During a one-month period, I read separate articles in the *New York Times*, and the Los Angeles *Times*, and *Newsweek* about women who had decided to have their breasts removed before they developed any signs of cancer.

The pros and cons of this controversial operation are more thoroughly discussed in the later chapter on reconstruction. However, one woman who chose this option and said she has no regrets is thirty-year-old Sharon Hughes of San Diego County. In a Los Angeles *Times* story, she said, "I knew I couldn't handle breast cancer mentally. And I didn't want to spend the next ten to fifteen years of my life worrying about it. I haven't regretted it at all." She explained she considered the surgery after biopsies had shown that her breast lumps contained atypical precancerous cells.

Newsweek reported that Carol Koch, a forty-four-year-old Sausalito, California, woman also had the procedure four years after her mother had been treated for breast cancer.

The operation is being recommended by a growing medical contingent for the woman who already has had cancer in one breast. The topic is frequently brought up when the woman is considering reconstruction for her mastectomy site. Recently, I heard one woman who had had breast cancer say that she had had her second breast removed for "peace of mind." During my last gynecological appointment, my doctor casually mentioned that one of his breast cancer patients had recently had a prophylactic mastectomy on her remaining breast.

The operation can be truly lifesaving, according to San Francisco plastic surgeon Vincent R. Pennisi, a long-time advocate of the procedure for moderate- and high-risk women. He said that in the course of performing subcutaneous mastectomies in his practice, he had found five totally unsuspected cancers and an additional five growths at the earliest stages of cancer development. In an earlier nationwide study he found eighty-two unsuspected cancers in a total of 1,385 women who had the surgery, a 6 percent incidence rate.

Pennisi admits that many of the women he operated on may never have developed breast cancer. But he believes that a wait-and-see attitude is "taking a big gamble." He explained, "I like to catch cancer before the fact, not after it has developed and already had time to spread."

It's a logical argument, but I wondered how many women were having their breasts amputated who would never develop breast cancer. The estimate, from Charles E. Horton, professor and chairman of plastic surgery at the Eastern Virginia Medical School, is as high as 85 percent. "But don't say we are removing the breasts unnecessarily," he added. "We're doing our best and we tell the woman she may never get breast cancer. These women know that they are sacrificing a breast with sexual stimulation, that they will have less feeling and that it won't look like their natural breast. But the risk is worth it to them. Some women worry about getting breast cancer so much that it ruins their lives."

"The problem is that we don't have good tests at the moment for telling who will and who won't get breast cancer," Horton explained. "All that we can tell the high-risk woman now is that in our estimate it's a good idea, because if you get breast cancer, you could die."

But another important concern was presented by surgeon Gordon F. Schwartz of the Jefferson Medical College in Philadelphia. In a paper presented at the 1981 Breast Cancer Conference, he said, "Without question, the manner in which risk is presented to the patient may make all the difference in her choice. If these women are made to understand the concept of risk, that a second cancer is not inevitable, there are very few who would not choose careful follow-up instead of a mastectomy. If, on the other hand, the likelihood of a subsequent cancer developing is made to sound inevitable, then a woman is more likely to succumb to the suggestion of prophylactic mastectomy."

Physicians have known about risk factors for decades, but only recently have they placed more value on their potential for controlling breast cancer. Some doctors already are analyzing your risk factors when you enter their office with a lump or even come in for a general and routine physical examination. But, it has to be noted that, for all its promise, there also is some risk in taking the information too seriously and in making irreversible decisions without really understanding what risk means or realizing researchers' still limited ability to predict who will and who will not develop breast cancer.

CHAPTER 4

Breast Cancer Psychology

Finding you have breast cancer is traumatic, not only because you must face all the fears that cancer can create, but also because the disease traditionally has led to coping with the loss of a breast. In the past, the medical community could understand why a woman would be upset about cancer, but couldn't understand why she would react so strongly to losing what one doctor called a "superficial, easily disposable appendage." The typical medical stance was, "Your life has been saved. What more could you want?" The woman who meekly replied, "My breast," or who reacted with prolonged tears or depression was at the least considered unappreciative and vain, and at worst possibly neurotic.

Today, medicine is doing a slow turnabout. Practitioners are placing new emphasis on the quality of life. They are also increasingly accepting the fact that many women see their breasts as a valued part of their bodies. It's difficult to think of another part of a woman's body that carries so much emotional symbolism. The message was clearly shown during a simple word association game at a training program for nurses on breast cancer. An instructor held up several pictures of breasts and asked women to describe their feelings in one-word responses. A woman gently nursing her baby brought responses of "security," "fulfillment," "warmth," "feminine," "beautiful," and "nurturing." A woman with a *Playboy*-sized cleavage evoked "arousal," "sensual," "beautiful," "assets," "pride," "bigger is better," but from other women came "ugly," "sex object," and "disgusting."

A partially nude woman advertising a pornographic movie got the most agreement: "sexist," "mindless," "exploitation." Next, a picture of a woman with a mastectomy: "sad," "loss," "fear," "death," but also "relief," "hope for cure," and "progress."

The replies show the range of emotional feelings about breasts and give clues to how personal and different the meaning of the breast can be for individual women. It's only natural for women to equate their femaleness and womanhood with breasts. Breast development is the first visible sign that they are leaving childhood behind and beginning to emerge into adult womanhood. Anthropologist Margaret Mead believed that the female breast has been so idealized in the United States that it is the woman's primary identification with the feminine role, in effect, a badge of femininity.

Some women seriously contend that the development or lack of development of their breasts has played an important role in their personality and lifestyle. One woman said, "Breasts were used by my peers as a sign of being more or less of a woman, of being mature. So my being flat meant that I was inferior, and it was used to ostracize me. I found myself on the fringe, not really knowing how to make friends. I was forced to turn inward. My prime concern became my work and my thoughts."

Another woman explained, "My heavy breasts made me inhibited and shy and physically restrained." Another said, "Having large breasts helped me think of myself as a sex symbol. Everyone else did. That attitude certainly didn't encourage me to do anything with myself intellectually. I never thought about having a career."

From time immemorial, women have used their breasts to reflect their opinions about themselves to others. In the 1920s, many women bound their breasts and slouched to achieve the flat-chested flapper look. In the 1940s and 1950s, women emphasized their femaleness with a little padding to help conform to role models like Marilyn Monroe, Jane Russell, and Rita Hayworth. "Bigger was definitely better," as far as breasts were concerned. Sex roles were carefully defined in culture and frequently outlined in "sweater girl" fashions. In the 1970s, breasts conveyed another message and many women went braless to declare their liberation and new-found freedoms.

With the help of consciousness-raising and the women's movement, women today are learning that their breasts do not define their value and role in society. Many women are demanding to be taken more seriously, pursuing and succeeding in careers that require high degrees of intelligence and ability. But that doesn't mean they don't want to be proud of their bodies.

Even with the positive advances made by the women's movement, we are still living in a breast-conscious society. For every person who buys the feminist-oriented *Ms.* magazine, five buy *Cosmopolitan* and twelve purchase *Playboy,* magazines whose editors believe that showing a woman with cleavage on the cover will help sales. That this is still a breast-conscious society is also evidenced by the fact that an estimated 300,000 women in the United States have had their breasts enlarged through surgery. About 30,000 to 40,000 women have this operation each year. Another 15,000 to 20,000 a year have their breasts reduced.

So much value has been placed on the breasts that just about every woman seems unhappy with her natural breast size, reports genetic counselor Patricia Kelly. She has talked with over 500 women about their feelings and less than a dozen were happy with their natural proportions. "Some complained that their breasts were too large. Others said their breasts were too small."

Society continues to send out conflicting messages. One woman told her, "I know my boyfriend says he will still love me if I get breast cancer, but then we go to a party and he measures women's attractiveness by their breast size."

Although not all cultures value breasts as sexual organs, they are a prime erogenous zone in American culture. About half of all women have been estimated to be sexually aroused by breast play. Nipples especially are highly sensitive to stimulation because their nerve endings are connected to the erogenous areas of the brain.

Some men and women still believe that the larger a woman's breasts the more excitable she is and that relatively flat-chested women have little interest in sex. Actually, nothing could be further from the truth. Sex therapists William H. Masters and Virginia E. Johnson write, "There is absolutely no evidence to suggest that breast size bears any relation to a woman's level of sexual interest, to her capacity for sexual response or to the ease with which she achieves orgasm." Their studies found that the woman who does become sexually excited when her breasts are stimulated does so regardless of their size. Whether breasts are responsive to stimulation or not, they are involved in most couples' sexual foreplay. It's no wonder that many women equate breast loss with a loss of sexual attractiveness.

Sex therapist Lonnie Barbach interviewed women who had had

mastectomies and found it common for many to feel unattractive and disfigured after surgery. She and other therapists believe that the problem is often magnified in the mind of the woman, but whether the problem is real or imagined, Barbach said most women have to come to terms with their new sexual identity. Most women do succeed, but it isn't always easy and it can take time. Many of the women she interviewed delayed having sexual intercourse for much longer than it took them to recover physically from their operation. A couple of women who have had mastectomies told me that they no longer enjoy sleeping in the nude and go to bed in flannel nightgowns.

It's easy to understand why breasts symbolize motherhood. Although women went through an era of feeding babies from bottles, many now know that the best formula comes from their own breasts. And although most women would never consider exposing their breasts in public under normal circumstances, it's not unusual to see a woman quietly nursing her baby in public. Breast-feeding is a natural and healthy experience. However, the link between the breasts and infants can create unexpected feelings in a young woman who has had a mastectomy and is thinking about pregnancy. One woman said, "I know I can have a baby, but somehow it doesn't seem right. The thought of me pregnant conjures up the Sunday paper cartoon that asks you to find the six things wrong with this picture. It's hard to imagine holding a baby against my plastic prosthesis or even getting up at night to the baby's cries and trying to comfort it against my concave chest."

Even without symbolic weight, breasts are important because they are a part of you, something you have grown up thinking is a normal and natural part of your body. Psychologists explain it a different way, saying that breasts are part of a woman's body image, quite simply, the way she sees herself in her own mind. Body image is often reflected in the way you project yourself to others. A person who thinks she is too tall, too fat, or too thin tends to project such feelings to other people.

Psychologist Wendy Schain, a medical health consultant for the National Institutes of Health, explains that feelings of self-worth or self-esteem are influenced by four major areas: the Body Self, which has a functional (what I can do) and an aesthetic (what I look like) part; an Interpersonal Self, which is influenced by friendships and social contacts as well as intimate and sexual contacts; the Achieving Self, which is based on elements of work or competitive efforts such as a good career or school achievements; and the Identification Self, which is made up of attitudes and behaviors related to spiritual, ethical, or ethnic concerns.

Schain explains that a loss in any of these areas can make a person feel devalued. For example, the severance of a long-term relationship may be seen as rejection or as an insult to the Interpersonal Self. But the person may compensate for the loss by borrowing good feelings or psychological stroking from the Body Self component, perhaps by working hard to develop a good figure. On the other hand, the child who is not considered attractive or who may not have an especially good personality may work very hard in school to become number one in order to compensate for not feeling adequate or worthwhile in the body image area of self-worth.

The crisis of cancer diagnosis can almost always be viewed as a threat to self-esteem and body image. U.C.L.A. nursing professor Sally Thomas agrees, noting that an amputation is a loss in terms of body image and integrity, no matter how lifesaving the operation may be.

One woman who had a mastectomy drew this parallel: "Obese people sometimes have difficulty in accepting their own bodies after having lost—willingly and deliberately—much weight. Imagine the distress of a woman who loses her breast against her will because of necessity . . . she has to adapt, almost overnight, to a radical change in her body image."

I'm not saying that a mastectomy is the worst fate that can befall a woman. Most women who get breast cancer say that fear of death and recurrence of cancer far outweigh their concern over breast loss. A study that asked women to rank the extent to which they would miss various parts of their body found that women would rather lose a breast than a tongue, a nose, an eye, a foot, an arm, or a hand. A little more than half the women responding to an American Cancer Society study in 1973 said that breast removal would make them "feel less of a woman," but an impressive 92 percent said they thought they could establish a normal life after a mastectomy.

What I am saying is that breast amputation is not and never should be taken lightly. A question I hear increasingly from women is that "If cancer of the penis were as common as cancer of the breast, would radical surgery be so common?'' Psychologist Beth E. Meyerowitz makes a similar comment in the February 1981 issue of *Professional Psychology*: "One might wonder if less mutilating treatments would have been developed and tested sooner if breast cancer weren't a 'woman's disease.'"

It's strange to read what psychologists consider a normal reaction to a crisis like breast cancer and compare it to my own feelings and reactions. Part of me is surprised when I hear women talk about how important breasts are and to hear them say that breast cancer is their worst fear. Part of me wants to say, "It's really not so bad." Yet another part knows I would be lying if I didn't admit that having breast cancer initially did affect my ego and feelings about my true worth. I think one thing I benefited from was never seeing myself as a real beauty when I was going through school. I chipped my front tooth in grade school and had to wear an obvious silver cap. Next came glasses, and although I had been underweight during early grade school years, I made up for it in eighth grade and through high school. My own sense of value came through being at least an average student and working as editor of my high school and college newspapers.

When I reached twenty-five, I was feeling pretty good about myself. I had graduated from college and had my first job as a reporter for a large urban paper. I dated several men, but really enjoyed my relationship with Jeff. I liked being a mature, adult woman, making decisions in my life, seeing what I could accomplish. I wasn't thinking about breast cancer. I felt that I had just run into a solid brick wall. That first year after my mastectomy, I felt as though I were taking a roller-coaster ride of emotions. There were new highs, when I would stop and realize how good it was to be alive, to feel the warmth of sunshine, to enjoy going to the zoo, taking a walk by the lake, or making a new recipe. The joy of still being here could come at the strangest times. There were new fears, like getting a knot in my stomach when I wrote an obituary for the paper and had to report cancer as the cause of death, and wondering the first time I was ill after my operation if all the discomfort and tiredness really came from the flu. And there were new lows, wondering whether I could have a good sexual relationship with any man or if anyone could still find me attractive, breaking into tears after seeing a woman with cleavage in a movie because I knew I could never look like that.

I remember, shortly after I returned to work, the news editor assigning me to write an in-depth series on the state's newly named Miss America—it was the first time a Wisconsin woman had won the title. "How could there be much depth to a beauty pageant winner," I, a budding feminist, mused. But the idea intrigued me, as I sat there, with one breast, trying to write a profile on the country's typical ideal woman. I threw myself into the story, if only to find out what made her so special.

Surprisingly, I ended up feeling better rather than worse about myself. For starters, I found a woman who wasn't a natural beauty, but who had built her own image, made herself attractive. And it hadn't been all that easy. She developed her singing ability while touring and performing with the folk group, the New Christy Minstrels. But before she could enter the beauty pageant, she had had to lose more than thirty pounds and worked to improve her speaking ability by volunteering to talk to grade-school children about her singing tours of Vietnam. She had spent hours at a modeling school learning to walk and to wear and coordinate clothes and an equal amount of time improving her voice and rehearsing the song she would sing in Atlantic City. She was special because she had made herself special. I'm glad I had that assignment, because I learned how much you can do with what you've got. I could see that my problem would be as bad as I chose to make it.

I decided again, "It's not so bad being me." Although I knew that I wouldn't make a very exciting find at a singles' bar, I had never gone to singles' bars anyway. I continued seeing several people, but still found Jeff the person I enjoyed most.

When I went back for my six-week checkup my doctor asked if I were married yet. I didn't know if he was joking or if he really meant that I should rush into marriage. I do know that getting married then would have been the very worst thing I could have done. It was important for me to realize that I was still the same person I had been before. Jeff and I had discussed getting married when he finished graduate school, and I wanted to stick to our plans, not change my life because a tumor had developed in my breast. It was important for me to know that Jeff wasn't marrying me out of a sense of obligation. The year's wait was good for both of us. I know some men would find it difficult to marry a woman without a breast, but he wasn't one of them. He took me seriously when I said that if he had any reservations about marrying somebody with breast cancer he would be doing me more harm than good by going through with the marriage. Although like any married couple we have had our disagreements and problems, they haven't been related to my having had breast cancer.

My feelings after my mastectomy were probably quite common. Psychologists write that just about every woman experiences some degree of depression, anxiety, and anger. In fact, many health professionals say their real concern is for a woman who doesn't show any signs of distress. Psychologist Netta Grandstaff sees a woman's emotional reactions as a normal part of the disease. She quotes psychotherapist Viktor Frankl: "There are things which cause you to lose your reason or you have none to lose. The abnormal reaction to the abnormal situation is normal behavior." I think it's important to list usual reactions following mastectomy, first because they are so rarely discussed by the medical community, and second because knowing that they are shared should prevent you from thinking that you are headed toward long-term serious mental disturbances if they do occur. Most women cope quite well and by the end of a year's time say their lives are back to normal. However, after surgery or a diagnosis of cancer, it's not unusual for women to show some signs of depression. Common symptoms include difficulty sleeping, changes in weight, changes in mood, recurrent nightmares, crying spells, difficulty in concentrating, difficulty in working, fatigue, and exhaustion. One woman told me, "All of a sudden I just started crying, for what then seemed like no apparent reason. For three days, I just kept crying."

When anger surfaces, it may be directed at the fact that you had a mastectomy ("Why me?") or displaced to the surgeon, nurses, hospital personnel, or family and friends. It may grow out of what happened to you or be triggered by your seeming lack of control or even at medical research, which has yet to come up with guarantees of cure.

When my surgeon entered my room the day after my mastectomy, I couldn't look at him. I felt he had betrayed me. I guess I still do. I clenched my fists, eyed the pitcher of water next to my bed, and decided that if I could hold back tears long enough I would dramatically tip the water over, at the same time telling him to get out of the room, that I wanted a different doctor and that I never wanted to see him again. I started counting backward—five-four-three—slowed down to wonder how long it would take the nurses to clean up the mess. I didn't want them around either. Then as I got to two, and the doctor started to describe the size of the tumor, his voice broke a little. I thought, "Well, either he has a cold or he didn't enjoy this experience any more than I did." I gave him the benefit of the doubt, although to this day I think it would have done me a world of good to have toppled that water pitcher.

In one study, women reported that their anxiety level was highest immediately after they discovered their lumps. Depression tended to pose the most difficult problem immediately after surgery and again two to three months following their operations. Many women reported that returning home after surgery wasn't especially upsetting. Some expressed guilt, thinking they might have caused their cancer to develop by something they did in life. For example, some fear, however irrationally, that they are being punished for masturbation or for premarital sex.

Otherwise normal and stable women may resort to denial, which can take many forms, from dropping the word *cancer* from your vocabulary to pretending you didn't really have the disease. It's common for women to say, "It's not really so bad"; "It was only a breast"; "You could hardly see it anyway."

Some believe that denial is an appropriate "emergency" tool for helping to maintain control and function normally in an extremely stressful situation. An article in the *Breast Cancer Digest* states, "Denial can serve as an emotional anesthetic; the threat is reduced, patients gradually can begin to absorb and deal with the reality of their situation until they feel strong enough to face all the problems and challenges that the disease and treatment pose."

While I was in the hospital after the mastectomy, my mother seemed distressed and Jeff seemed to be losing weight because he couldn't eat much. Everybody was waiting for my laboratory tests to come back to show whether the cancer had spread to the lymph nodes or other areas. When the doctor reported the good news that there was no evidence of spread, Jeff let out a sigh of relief. My mother seemed overjoyed. Their reactions truly surprised me. It's strange, but I never worried about spread. I didn't even consider it a possibility. For those few days, I felt I had total control over every single cell in my body. It was a wonderful feeling of power. I've rarely felt the same degree of control since. I suppose psychologists would call that stage denial. Maybe they are right. But it was such a strong feeling, I some-times wonder if it helped my own natural defenses against the disease.

NBC News correspondent Betty Rollin wrote a painfully frank and intimate description of her "crazy period" after her mastectomy. Many women I've talked to, and I myself, have been offended by her reactions. She sobbed, raged against the doctors who had misdiagnosed her lump, felt like a freak, cried some more, made outlandish remarks at parties, left her husband, moved in with somebody else, ended that relationship. I'm beginning to suspect, however, that part of the reason we resented her reaction was that it struck a raw nerve. Most women and men in today's society have been conditioned to be fairly passive and to deny their emotions. Women are only now being told that it's all right to "open up" and to "talk about one's feelings." In fact, it has been stated that the pendulum for breast cancer has swung from a medical view that dictated women should not be upset to a mental health view that says all women should be extremely upset. I think it's good that more support groups are available to women and that they are told they don't have to keep their feelings bottled inside. But the individuality of women needs to be kept in perspective, and, as psychologist Beth Meyerowitz says, not every woman should be ex-pected to "get in touch" with her emotional despair. Above all, women are individuals and should be able to design their own ways of coping. Meyerowitz stresses that the fact that some patients may use denial should never be an excuse to withhold information. Studies show that women who receive information about treatment options cope con-siderably better with their problems than those who feel they have no choice. A key cause of depression is a general feeling of helplessness. Withholding information and making a woman feel she has no control over her life is a sure way to encourage depression.

Studies are few and mostly anecdotal, but some guidelines may help in understanding why every woman copes differently. How those you have known with breast cancer have responded to treatment may influence your optimism or lead to more anxiety and pessimism. For example, one woman whose sister lived less than a year after her mas-tectomy found it extremely difficult to view her future optimistically, even though she had an excellent prognosis. Another woman, whose mother, despite breast cancer, had lived out a normal lifetime, had the opposite reaction.

The woman with a mastectomy who has accepted the view that her worth is defined by her appearance and physical attributes may find breast loss devastating, a true threat to her feelings of self-worth and femininity. It will probably be more difficult for her to adapt to her surgery than for the woman whose feelings of value are linked to achievement, intelligence, personality, or family life.

Psychologists believe that a model, a dancer, an athlete, or any woman whose career is dependent on maintaining a flawless or well-maintained body, may also have greater difficulty accepting breast loss.

There is disagreement over whether breast loss is harder for the younger or the older woman. Again, one can't generalize. My own feeling is that it can be just as devastating for the older as for the younger woman. Older women, however, are heavily conditioned by society not to be concerned about their appearance or body after a certain age. A fairly sensitive and intelligent doctor told me he didn't think that a breast was as important to older women. In this case, I think he was using denial. One fifty-six-year-old woman who was interested in reconstruction was actually asked by her doctor, "Now why would you want that? Whom are you going to seduce?"

Los Angeles psychiatrist Marcia Goin interviewed twelve women interested in reconstruction whose ages ranged from forty-five to sixty-five. Outwardly, she said, the women coped beautifully, but interviews began to uncover continuing feelings of loss, depression, and shame about sexual desires they believed were inappropriate for their age. Goin explained that our culture tends to repress the fact that older women have sexual feelings and denies that they might care about breast loss.

She said that five of the women still showed signs of depression, but it was typical for them to think of their depression as "disgusting feelings of self-pity." Although they had had moments of sadness, and crying spells, they gave in to these only when they were alone. Sexual desire decreased or disappeared; they considered it ludicrous to think of themselves as sexually desirable. One woman felt embarrassed about seeking reconstruction saying, "These things aren't supposed to matter to a woman my age."

Goin advises, "Physicians should be alert to their own prejudices that may influence them to accept things at face value," and asks, "Wouldn't we all like to believe that life gets easier as we get older and that then we can more easily accept losses and physical deterioration?"

When you are coping with breast cancer, it's impossible to divorce your reaction from other events in your life. For example, a newly married young woman with a good job and a loving husband may have a far easier time facing up to breast cancer than a middle-aged woman who has just learned that her husband is having an affair. A doctor expanded "Are you happy with your current job?" "Are your children doing well?" "Are your friends doing well?"—all can make a difference in how well a woman reacts to and copes with her disease.

Other key factors are the stage of your illness, whether you have radiation and chemotherapy, and your support system. Chemotherapy and radiation may delay emotional recovery, and many women go through mild depression right at the end of their treatment.

I know how valuable support can be. Even if Jeff and I had never married, his being at the hospital telling me that he loved me made my adjustment much easier than if I had had to go through the experience alone. I was fortunate. I know that everybody isn't so lucky. One woman told me, "My boyfriend stopped in the day after my mastectomy for five minutes. I never saw him after that. It wasn't as though he had to marry me," she said, "but it would have been nice to have somebody there to hold my hand, to tell me how well I was doing."

Support can also come from family, friends, and relatives. Although my first choice was to keep my surgery a secret, I was happy that the word got out, for the letters and flowers and visits from people I cared about were a real boost to my morale.

A bonus can come from having doctors and nurses who take you seriously. I think it's reasonable to expect your doctor to give you good technical care, outline options, give you his or her suggestions, but also let you make your own decisions. Problems have developed in the past when doctors imposed their values and judgments on women, but also because women placed their doctors on pedestals as caretakers and great humanitarians. I think it's unrealistic to expect doctors to solve your problems, to get involved in your life or to put your expectations above their own personal concerns. However, their exhibiting a little warmth and compassion can certainly help and it often doesn't take that much extra effort.

Barbara, a young woman from Berkeley, said she had to consult with several doctors following her mastectomy. Each asked why she was there. "Breast cancer," she answered. Later she said, "Their reaction was the same as if I had just spelled my last name." Finally, when she went through the procedure for the fourth time, a doctor looked up and said, "Oh, I'm sorry." "That really made a difference," said Barbara.

Eve, a middle-aged woman from Oakland, reviewed her recent treatment for breast cancer and said that one of the worst things a doctor can do is make you feel you are overreacting. Her radiation therapist, obviously upset when Eve became depressed halfway through her treatment sessions, tried to tell her how lucky she was. "I exploded," said Eve. "Look, I know how lucky I am. I only have to look around at the other patients receiving radiation to know that I'm one of the fortunate ones. But, this is my disease and I really didn't want anybody else telling me how lucky I am."

I had similar feelings when I saw my doctor after my failed reconstruction and he said I was lucky I had only had an implant removed. "Think how much worse it would have been if you had had the more involved procedure and that hadn't worked. Then it would have been a real disaster." I would have appreciated a little compassion at that time. Even when you have a common cold, it's nice not to be told how fortunate you are that you only have a cold.

Women who have been through the same experience can be an important resource. I know doctors who don't like Reach to Recovery volunteers to visit their patients. Reasons given are that the doctors think the group is like a club or that they themselves can provide all the support the woman needs. I think a patient should at least be asked if she would like to talk to someone who has been through the experience. It is good to talk with somebody who has had chemotherapy or radiation if that is what you're scheduled to receive. You get the luck of the draw in the individual woman you get to talk to, but I think it's worth the effort. Contact may be especially helpful in today's highly mobile society where it's not unusual to find women living in a different state from relatives and where divorce and being single are increasing trends.

Some problems affect almost all cancer patients. One is a tendency to overreact to the slightest ailment. A cold, a sore throat, even easy weight loss may suddenly reactivate the anxiety you felt when you discovered your lump. Many women report having occasional relapses of sadness and depression. A number of unexpected events can re-awaken the original fears and concerns over having cancer or over breast loss. Death of others from cancer, newspaper articles that describe cancer treatment, and new clothes that reveal the incision are a few of the subtle catalysts that may touch off feelings and fears, according to one psychologist. The worst time for me was after my reconstruction failure. The experience recalled my mastectomy; it was almost like losing a breast a second time, something I hadn't expected. That was probably the only time that I suffered serious depression, but even that eased as I forced myself to get involved in activities. I tried to take a message from Sherry, a lovely middle-aged woman who discussed her ups and downs with breast cancer on a videotaped interview available from the American Cancer Society. Looking back on her mastectomy and still undergoing a program of chemotherapy, she advised, "Keeping busy is the secret of not getting depressed." Sherry added, "You have to make a conscious effort to reach down inside yourself to say you're going to enjoy today." Still, another difficult time was when a friend—a colleague who worked in the next office —died of cancer. Although he had my deepest concern and sympathy, I also had to ask myself if I were looking into a mirror. I found myself losing weight and went to a doctor to have a swollen node in my throat checked. My anxiety probably wasn't unusual. I have had other friends die of cancer since then but my reaction hasn't been so intense, if only because I understand my true fears and can deal better with them.

Another common concern is what to tell your children and when. Psychologists seem agreed that truthfulness is the best policy. The unknown is often more frightening than facts, and a child may imagine a situation worse than reality. If you're reluctant to tell a child, your doctor or a social worker or counselor may be able to help you explain that you are having treatment for breast cancer. Some counselors say that this may be an especially difficult time for a teenage daughter who identifies closely with her mother and wonders whether she too will get breast cancer. Again, knowing that this may be an issue could help you sit down and discuss it with her or find someone with whom she can discuss her worry.

On the issue of sexuality, I think every woman has to make some kind of a sexual adjustment, but again, from my own experience and from listening to other women, I know that most women do adjust.

The few studies that have been conducted tend to show that if you had a good sexual relationship before a mastectomy, your chances are excellent for having a good sexual relationship afterward. Some couples report that learning to be more sensitive to each other's needs can make the experience even better. However, if you were having problems before your mastectomy, it would be a disservice for anyone to tell you that your marriage will improve after having breast cancer. The simple facts are that there is an adjustment to be made, you have to come to terms with your new self, and it does take time. One study found that one third of women were still having sexual problems one year after mastectomy. In this breast-conscious society, it is again easy to understand why.

I think you have to be ready to acknowledge that some men will not be able to accept a relationship with a woman with one breast. However, I think it's time to turn the table and take a suggestion from sex therapist Bernie Zilbergeld, who in his book *Male Sexuality*, offered advice to men on what to do if they ran into a woman who measured them by inches. "Just as there are a few men who will absolutely not have sex with a woman unless her breasts can fill a 38-D bra, there are probably a few women who won't be satisfied with anything less than a twelve-inch penis. Should it be your misfortune to run into one of these women, the only reasonable suggestion we can make is that you get away as quickly as possible. Being that concerned about a physical characteristic over which no one can have any control is not a good sign. Besides if you don't have the requisite number of inches there is nothing you can do about it. Better to spend your time with one of the millions of women who couldn't care less about such things."

Yes, some men won't want to have sexual relations with a woman who has had a mastectomy, but I am convinced that women tend to overestimate the number. Some men don't like fat women; some don't like skinny ones. Some don't like assertive women; some dislike the unassertive. If you try to please every man, you're headed for trouble.

The 1980 technical report for the National Cancer Institute contained two questions aimed at determining men's reactions to breast loss. The first question asked men to imagine how a single man's physical attraction might change to a woman who had to have a breast removed. Three times as many men said the situation definitely would be more difficult than dealing with a woman who had had a hysterectomy. Only 5 percent said they thought the man would find the woman "much less attractive." Fifty-one percent replied that the man would find the woman "just as attractive as before the operation," and 35 percent replied that the woman would be "somewhat less attractive." If they themselves were faced with the situation, 44 percent of the men said they would love their wife or partner just the same, that the breast removal would make no difference. Thirty-seven percent said they would have sympathy, compassion, support for her, and stand beside her, and 18 percent said they would "be glad she's alive." Another 18 percent said they "would be upset, concerned, sorrowful, and have personal sadness." Even if this study underestimates the reactions of men to breast loss, it still leaves a lot of eligible men around.

Sex therapist Lonnie Barbach points out that it's only normal for a man to have to come to terms with the mastectomy site. Initially, looking at the site can be a shock, just as it is for the woman. Half the battle is being able to look at the scar yourself and see that it's not as bad as feared. She advises a woman with a mastectomy to examine her scar, look at herself in the mirror, touch, examine, and become familiar with the area. She gave an example from a therapy session she conducted for women who were having difficulty achieving orgasm. The session included Beth, a woman who had had a mastectomy. As the group exchanged more information, Beth admitted that she had had her breast removed and still had difficulty talking about it. The other women, who had never seen a mastectomy scar, asked to see it. Beth reluctantly took off her blouse and her prosthesis, and the women looked at her chest, touched it, examined it. They agreed that it didn't look as bad as they had expected. "It was a turning point for the woman," said Barbach. "She had felt really alone and wretched and thought she had something to hide that would repulse anyone who saw it."

Communication is for many the key to developing and maintaining a good sexual and marital relationship. Once you air your fears and feelings, a man has a chance to respond. If you don't communicate, you will be increasing your chances of problems and misunderstandings.

Lynn described her experiences with her husband, Charles, in an article for *Good Housekeeping* magazine. After she left the hospital, he tried to give her a big hug. "I pulled away because my incision was still tender," she said. "From then on, he went out of his way to avoid touching me. Even if he accidentally brushed against me, he'd back off.

But the most obvious change was in bed. We always used to hold each other close before going to sleep even if we had no intention of making love. Now, he gave me a perfunctory kiss, pressed my hand briefly, and moved to his side of the bed."

Lynn said she felt it reasonable that her husband didn't want an incomplete woman. She continued, "That's when I started to hide myself from Charles. I wore baggy flannel nightgowns and changed clothes behind doors. I avoided physical contact with him and I'd either go to bed before him or stay up much later reading. It was less painful than being rejected." Lynn said she later met a woman in her doctor's office who had been married only six months but had had a mastectomy two years previously and was checking to find if it were O.K. to get pregnant.

"Do you mean you got married after your operation?" she asked. The woman picked up the surprise and said, "You sound as though you don't think a woman could appeal to a man sexually because she'd lost a breast. Some men might feel like that, but I doubt many would. Sexual attraction rests on a lot more than a breast."

Later that night Lynn told her husband about the encounter and asked "Can you imagine, a man marrying a woman who's had a mastectomy?" "What's so strange about that?" Charles replied. "A man doesn't fall in love with a part of a woman's body. He falls in love with the whole woman." Lynn asked why he had been drawing away from her for weeks. "I thought I disgusted you," said Lynn. "I was afraid I might hurt you. I didn't know when it would be all right to hold you, to caress you, to make love to you. I was waiting for you to tell me," Charles said.

I've known too many women who have had mastectomies and have good marital relationships and too many women who have married or had love affairs after their mastectomies to think that a woman has to forget about sex when she loses a breast.

If you're single, you're faced with special concerns. Alice, a divorced woman with two children, explained that there is a problem of when to tell the man you're dating that you have had a mastectomy. She explained in a brief chapter she wrote in the book *Decision for Life*, "I'm not the kind of person to get involved right away. That would be too threatening. I have to know the person. The fact of my mastectomy is not a big problem for me now. My only concern is, when is the right time to tell someone about it? I've decided that it's after you've known a person for a while and can see he has an interest in you, and you are interested in him. You shouldn't wait until you're ready to go to bed. You have to tell him at some discreet time before-hand when you know that something could develop."

Barbach said that, to a large extent, the problem of a mastectomy will be as big as you make it. "How you handle a situation determines the results you'll get." She gives an example of counseling women in wheelchairs with shriveled legs. "Those who are self-conscious and withdrawn tend to appear unattractive. But the woman who is warm and outgoing invites social contacts. You can't underestimate what you can do with yourself."

One therapist, who has had two mastectomies, advises, "Don't be afraid to try, become more aware of your sexual feelings and needs, read sex manuals, talk about sex with your partner; don't be afraid to explore and expand."

And from an oncologist, "You can achieve sexual satisfaction with or without a breast, but it certainly helps to start feeling good about yourself. You can learn to be more seductive, arouse a man to a higher state so that he just wants you as a person. That's probably the simplest technique."

Another sex therapist, who has had two mastectomies herself, suggests that a woman may want to conjure up some interesting under-wear or a nightgown and camouflage the mastectomy site until she is ready to disrobe and let her partner see or touch the wound area.

Every woman has to find her own way of coping. Change takes courage, but the only way to find out what will happen is to try. I also believe that radiation therapy and reconstruction are two new options that can make the process easier for many women. Another positive advantage of these procedures is that the fear of death and recurrence that many women live with after having cancer can be decreased. One woman whose radiation therapy left her with a near normal breast told me, "Cancer seemed just a stage in my life." It's not uncommon for women who have had reconstruction to say that they like the improvement if only because breast loss is no longer a conspicuous daily reminder that they had cancer. I think it's harder for many women with a missing breast to adopt such a positive attitude.

Psychologist Schain explains that the more conservative pro-cedures and breast reconstruction can help preserve your body, but,

"You still have the medical status that you had before. However," she says, "if forgetting that you had cancer or downplaying its importance is a type of rationalization that minimizes depression and does not interfere with good health maintenance, then I support it as a protective and not destructive manner of coping."

Breast cancer is a crisis in life, and it takes untapped strength to deal with it. Although Reach to Recovery volunteers tell women that they are the same person they were before the operation, I tend to disagree. For some, life will be worse. But many women who do cope with the disease find themselves stronger, more self-assured, and capable of leading more fulfilling lives. If you've gone through the crisis of breast cancer, you can go through just about anything.

"I consider every day a very precious gift," twenty-eight-year-old Sheila Jackson said. "I'm probably not as willing to compromise and give up what I want to do. I think I use my time more constructively, too. Another thing, I'm not very tolerant when I hear people complain about how they look, about being overweight, or maybe about having to take care of young children. I'm not going to listen until they complain about something they have no control over." She adds, "I really think there is more depth to my personality and emotions."

Another woman echoed this message. "I have changed gradually, but dramatically. The change began the day I decided, 'The time I have left, I'm going to use well,' and began to rearrange my priorities and look at myself and my life in a more positive way. I used to live only for my family. My family is meaningful to me, but I'm meaningful to me now too. I'm just as important as other people—and that's a big part of the change. I no longer get inundated with things that don't interest me. I'm learning to say no, whereas before I wondered what people would have thought of me if I had said that. And I no longer give a darn what the neighbors think. Before my mastectomy I went through each day thinking I was immortal. Now I only want to live each day positively. I don't want to waste my energies in negativism. I know where I am because I had to face it. And I can never go back."

California Chief Justice Rose Bird, writing about her 1976 encounter with breast cancer and subsequent recurrences, said, "If I had not come to terms with the possibility of my own death and my own mortality, if I had not been able to face the fact that I had cancer and to face the fears that cancer creates, I would have been devastated by many of my everyday experiences.

"About one week after my third operation was in the press, one of my most vocal critics began to make public speeches about the importance of getting rid of the 'cancer' at the top of the court. I was able to keep some perspective and even my sense of humor about it precisely because I had come to terms with my disease. Have courage, face the facts, and you will find that when you have faced your fears and stood your ground there occurs a kind of liberation. It is not an easy journey. It can be quite painful and lonely. But it is a journey that must be made. It is not a hopeless situation. It is neither too painful nor too fearful to face. Most important, it is an opportunity to find out about life. And isn't that really why each of us has been placed here?"

CHAPTER 5

Where Are We Today?

Today, it's unusual not to know at least one person who has had breast cancer. You mention the disease, and you hear about Bob's wife or Judy's aunt who just had a breast removed. You pick up the paper and read that a well-known actress has just had an operation—"the modified kind"—and former President Carter's mother, Miss Lillian, had a breast operation at the age of eighty-two.

It's not your imagination—more women than ever before are being treated for breast cancer in the United States. Some 112,000 women are expected to get breast cancer in 1982. The number is a drastic increase from even only four years ago, when 107,000 women were treated. In 1970, the number was just 69,000.

Contrary to what you may think, the country is not in the middle of a breast cancer epidemic. Incidence rates per 100,000 population have increased by only about 2 percent a year in the 1970s, well behind rates of lung, skin, and uterine cancer in women.

Most of the increase in breast cancer cases is explained by population growth in the United States, especially among older women, the group most vulnerable to breast cancer. Women sixty-five and older comprise the fastest growing segment of the U.S. population. Between 1960 and 1970, their number increased by 41 percent, and predictions for the year 2035 are that the number of women in this category will more than double. Clearly, the problem will only increase in the years ahead.

Aside from age, possible explanations for the higher rate of breast cancer include increased fat and meat consumption, changing patterns in the age of having children and the possibility that new diagnostic procedures are detecting more borderline cases of cancer, and perhaps overdiagnosing some cases that aren't cancer.

Several doctors I've talked to say they are seeing more young women with breast cancer, but so far their individual experiences can't be backed up by changes in national statistics.

I've only read about one man who had breast cancer. At first, he complained about feeling uncomfortable at the beach, not knowing quite what to do about the scar across his chest and his missing nipple. He eventually got as tan as anybody, thinking that the scar gave him an air of distinction. This man was among the 1,000 men a year who get the disease. It's unusual, but breast cancer does occur in men.

In fact, the first reference to breast cancer, describing "bulging tumors" in male breasts, was made some 3,000 years before Christ. The information is inscribed in hieroglyphiclike script on thin sheets of papyrus, possibly by the first known physician, the Egyptian Imhotep. The learned physician stated quite accurately, "There is no treatment."

The father of medicine, Hippocrates, born in Greece in 460 B.C., was equally pessimistic about treating patients with cancer. He wrote, "It is better not to apply any treatment . . . for if treated, the patients die quickly; but if not treated, they hold out for a long time."

Throughout the centuries various remedies were tried. They ranged from the application of "caustics," arsenic or zinc chloride paste, to the use of live frogs or chickens cut in half and laid on the breast. The physician to Queen Elizabeth I, William Clowes (1560–1634) believed that the "laying on of hands" could bring about a cure, and the good Elizabeth reportedly touched thousands in hope that their disease would thereby disappear. William A. Cooper, in his history of mastectomy adds, "And Clowes no doubt was as near the truth as was James Cooke who a few years later advised bleeding . . . or Peter Lowe who in 1597, was suggesting the application of goat's dung." Cures during any age were few. In fact, one historian wrote that "most cancers that were reported as cured probably were not cancers."

The French surgeon Jean Louis Petit (1674–1750) is credited with introducing the modern era of breast surgery. Although his "Traité des Opérations" was not published until twenty-four years after his death, his teachings became widely known in the 1720s through the surgical texts of contemporaries. Petit emphasized curing, rather than just removing, the cancer. He believed that the roots of the disease originated in the lymph nodes under the arm. A cancer operation, he contended, should be certain to remove these nodes. And rather than leave behind disease, he also suggested removing some of the chest muscles. However, whenever possible, he preserved the nipple and part of the breast not involved with cancer.

But this was years before the advent of anesthesia in 1846 and antiseptic surgery in 1867. Few patients survived any operation. As late as the early nineteenth century, the death rate was fully 95 percent for operations of the hip and 70 to 80 percent for thigh operations. In even the best clinics, 25 percent of women died during or shortly after breast cancer surgery. As late as the 1870s, survival rates at three years ranged between 5 and 20 percent, and cancers reappeared in many women's mastectomy sites before their wounds had even healed. No wonder many doctors advised against treatment, calling it both rash and cruel. Sir James Paget, lecturing on surgical pathology in 1853, said, "I do not despair of carcinoma being cured somewhat in the future, but this blessed achievement will never be wrought by the knife of the surgeon."

Despite Paget's misgivings, the most profound and long-lasting contribution to breast cancer treatment was soon to come from a new type of surgery introduced by William Stewart Halsted (1852–1922). A professor of surgery at Johns Hopkins University, he felt it important to routinely remove a woman's entire breast, as many lymph nodes as possible, and at least one of her two chest muscles. The operation, with some modifications, remained the treatment of choice for American surgeons into the early 1970s.

Although many modern women may feel that Halsted should have been burned at the stake for his impact on breast surgery, the fact is that nothing had produced better results. Reading his memorial tribute and a review of his many contributions shows him to be a truly remarkable and compassionate physician. "Dr. Halsted's gentleness and kindness, his great concern for suffering, his minute precautions against the unnecessary spilling or waste of blood, his watchfulness and anxiety about the fate of patients, afford one of the most touching and beautiful examples of humanity and the humane qualities of the real surgeon." The eulogy was delivered at Halsted's memorial in 1923 by surgery professor Rudolph Matas, one of the many who placed Halsted and his accomplishments on a pedestal. Others called him "one of the greatest surgeons of his generation."

Halsted seems to have been a fascinating and likable man, but he was as capable of making mistakes as any person. A medical journal from his own university hospital outlined both his successes and problems, noting that the Halsted family lived in New York and was prominent financially and active in various philanthropic projects. Young Halsted entered Yale at eighteen, but his scholastic record was poor. He never borrowed any books from the Yale library; he elected to spend most of his time at various types of athletics. In his senior year, he was captain of Yale's football team.

He continued studying at the College of Physicians and Surgeons in New York, where he developed an intense interest in anatomy, and graduated with honors in 1877. During the next two years, he studied anatomy in Europe where he learned firsthand about antiseptic surgery. On his return to New York in 1880, he helped establish the first surgical outpatient department in Bellevue Hospital. Around this time he became fascinated with the discovery that the cornea of the eye could be anesthetized with cocaine. By experimenting on himself he found that injecting the drug into a sensory nerve could make the whole area insensitive to pain, a finding that was soon applied to dental practice. Later Halsted discovered how to block the spinal cord with anesthetic drugs.

He didn't know, when he began experimenting on himself, that cocaine was habit-forming. An article in the *Johns Hopkins Medical Journal* recounts that although he overcame his addiction, the episode radically changed his whole life. He returned to New York after his cure to a more thoughtful and leisurely existence, with time for reflection and study of the surgical problems that interested him most. His life was far more fruitful than it could have been if he had continued the strenuous pace he had set for himself in the beginning.

Halsted investigated new surgical techniques, studied the healing patterns of wounds, recommended using fine silk rather than catgut for closing incisions, and developed successful techniques for skin grafts. His group is credited with being the first in the country to routinely use rubber gloves in surgery, but not to avoid spreading infection. Rather, Halstead had thin rubber gloves designed after his surgical nurse complained that the harsh operating room solutions irritated her arms and hands.

In 1890, Halsted published a summary of thirteen cases of breast cancer he had treated by his original technique of radical mastectomy.

He reported: "About eight years ago [1882] I began not only to typically clean out the axilla [armpit area] in all cases of cancer of the breast but also to excise in almost every case the pectoralis major [chest] muscle, or at least a generous piece of it, and to give the tumor on all sides an exceedingly wide berth."

In a later article, Halsted wrote that he frequently had to close his wide incisions with skin grafts from the patient's thigh. But, he said, "It is better to remove too much skin than too little, for the mistake of excising an insufficient quantity is quite fatal to the patient's chances of recovery."

He explained elsewhere: "Disability, ever so great, is a matter of very little importance as compared with the life of the patient. Furthermore, these patients are old. Their average age is nearly 55 years. They are no longer very active members of society. [I wonder if he would say the same about today's fifty-year-old women?] We should, perhaps, sacrifice many lives if we were to consider the disability which might result from removing a little more tissue here and there."

Other doctors had allowed only fifteen to twenty minutes for a breast operation, but Halsted's process could take four hours. He rarely performed more than one breast operation a day. His whole theory rested on the premise that cancer could be caught and cured if it were removed before it spread beyond the lymph nodes and chest muscles. When patients died, he felt it was because his operation had not been radical enough. At one point, Halsted advocated removing nodes in the neck, but later abandoned the practice as too drastic. He was quick to criticize doctors who refused to send patients to surgeons and who believed that cancer could not be cured. "We can state positively that cancer of the breast is a curable disease if operated upon properly and in time," he wrote in one of his early papers.

Halsted indeed had impressive statistics to report, as among his first fifty patients, only 6 percent had local recurrences in the chest area. Surgeons using other techniques had 60 to 80 percent recurrence rates.

A 1908 report based on more than 200 women documented that three-year survival rates for women without signs of spread to lymph nodes climbed to 85 percent. It was an impressive record, and the procedure spread as gospel among American surgeons.

Only ten days after Halsted presented his first formal paper on his treatment of breast cancer, Willy Meyer of New York presented a similar technique before the New York Academy of Medicine. Meyer's closing stitch went into the arm. His surgery did not remove as much skin as Halsted's procedure, but did remove both chest muscles. Ironically, although the radical mastectomy was to bear Halsted's name, the technique adopted by most surgeons was Meyer's procedure.

Once the radical mastectomy was established, it was hard for surgeons to retreat. As one surgery professor explained: "The radical mastectomy was quickly accepted because survival and local recurrence rates were unquestionably better than what anything else had been able to produce. Results were attributed to the extensive operation and it was hard for many to do any less."

He explained that what had been forgotten was that other major advancements, which also made a big impact on survival and local recurrence rates, had come at roughly the same time. Anesthesia was by then generally available. Antiseptics had arrived to cut down infection. When Halsted first designed the operation, he was often treating women whose tumors he described as "taking up the entire breast," or the size of "an orange," "a hen's egg," " a duck's egg."

The physician's charismatic personality and more humane techniques encouraged women to seek advice earlier, when their lesions were smaller. Halsted wrote, "Patients frequently come to us of their own accord against the will of their doctor." All of his early patients had obvious signs of disease spread, but by 1907 he could report that nearly 25 percent of his patients did not have disease in their lymph nodes.

It took close to half a century before anyone dared to question his operation. The early critics were considered heretics.

The first break with tradition came from Great Britain. Sir Geoffrey Keynes reported excellent results on some 200 patients treated, up to 1937, by local removal of the tumor and radium needle implants, although the outbreak of the war in 1939 brought an end to this important study. Immediately after World War II, Professor Robert McWhirter of Edinburgh reported good results on patients treated by removing only the breast (simple mastectomy) followed by radiotherapy. He found no difference between the length of survival of patients in his series and those who had been subjected to radical mastectomy.

England benefited from an early emphasis on carefully designed studies of treatments. Hundreds of women were randomly sorted into groups receiving different care and then watched to learn if one group did better than any other. The outcome showed that conservative methods of treatment resulted in survival rates similar to those obtained by radical, mutilating surgery. Indeed, by 1969, a survey of surgical practice in the United Kingdom found a marked swing away from radical surgery to more conservative operations (the simple mastectomy and radiotherapy or the modified radical mastectomy) that did not remove the chest muscles.

One woman told me of a friend who was living in Paris ten years ago when she discovered a breast lump. "Would you believe it?" she asked. "She was only treated with a lumpectomy, where they just remove the tumor, and radiate the breast."

I wasn't surprised, because doctors in many countries have been years ahead of the United States in switching to less radical procedures. A major 1981 *Consumer Reports* article on radiation notes that in France and in parts of Canada, where the procedure was pioneered, surgery is losing out to the lumpectomy and modern radiation therapy. The article quotes Roy M. Clark, a senior radiation oncologist at Princess Margaret Hospital in Toronto, as saying, "I think in ten years you won't see mastectomies performed here for early breast cancer."

Ironically, at the time surgeons in other countries were switching to less radical treatments, the doctors in the United States were not only firmly entrenched in performing radical mastectomies, but some were suggesting a more extensive operation—the extended radical mastectomy. This operation removed all that was excised in the radical mastectomy, plus lymph nodes under the chest bone; sometimes a portion of the rib cage would have to be removed. This procedure was done during the 1950s and 1960s by surgeons who were trying to remove as many lymph nodes as possible. The operation had a high complication rate and fortunately has been virtually abandoned since studies showed that it did nothing to improve survival rates.

One of the first voices in the United States to plead for both patients' rights and less radical surgery was George Crile, Jr., a surgeon at the Cleveland Clinic. Twelve percent of his patients received a partial mastectomy as early as 1955, and the radical mastectomy was discontinued for all patients at his clinic by 1957.

Crile considered the radical mastectomy to be "archaic" and said it had no place in the modern treatment of breast cancer. His own suggestion: "In case of doubt, accept the treatment that involves the least deformity, discomfort, disability, and risk of fatal complications." Crile's first wife had a simple mastectomy, but died from breast cancer. His second wife. Helga, discovered a very small lump, less than one half inch in diameter (1 cm), while having a routine mammogram in 1974 and had a partial mastectomy.

However, others called Crile's beliefs, "a great leap backwards in the treatment of carcinoma of the breast." Noted pathologist and surgeon C. D. Haagensen of Columbia University wrote in a 1973 editorial in the *Journal of the American Medical Association*, "The truth is that we already know enough regarding the inferiority of lumpectomy and the simple mastectomy . . . to conclude that it is not wise or humane to condemn a woman to be treated with these methods. Physicians who do should recall that Rabelais long ago said, 'Science without conscience is but ruination of the soul.'"

At the time Haagensen wrote his editorial, some doctors were beginning to change, but a good 50 percent supported him and continued to routinely perform the radical mastectomy. It wasn't until 1979 when policy officially changed in the United States. At that time, the National Institutes of Health invited international experts to attend a Consensus Development Conference to debate the best treatment for early breast cancer. The recommendation was that the radical operation should be set aside because other less mutilating surgery offered the same survival rates without the complications.

Radical mastectomy can result in a sunken chest wall, frequent swelling of the arm because so many lymph nodes (which normally help remove fluid) have been removed, and possible shoulder stiffness. A sixty-year-old Oakland school teacher who has lived with her radical mastectomy for ten years describes other problems. "I've adjusted to having had a mastectomy and don't think it affected any of my activities. The only problem is that I'm limited in the clothes that I can wear. I usually wear dresses that have long sleeves and a high neckline. When I buy clothes, I can't really look for ones that I like. I buy ones that fit. Sometimes in the dressing room, I just want to scream and tear the clothes off. But it's something I live with and keep to myself."

The 1979 consensus group advocated that the new treatment of choice for early breast cancer should be a total mastectomy with a separate incision (an axillary dissection) made under the armpit to remove lymph nodes. Although many label today's new standard a modified radical mastectomy, the National Institutes of Health states that "total mastectomy with axillary dissection" is the correct and preferred terminology. A key difference between the two operations is that the modified radical mastectomy removes the breast and nodes with one continuous incision. The new choice does it with two smaller incisions that give better cosmetic results to the patient.

Today, most doctors feel that it is only necessary to perform a radical mastectomy in the small number of cases where a tumor is growing directly into the chest muscles. Other doctors say even then it may be possible to remove only part of the chest muscles. They also know that if a radical has to be performed the operation does not have to sacrifice as much skin as was advocated by Halsted and that lymph nodes can be removed with an inconspicuous incision running under the armpit instead of one that goes high into the shoulder area and continues down into the arm.

A major study, which convinced many that radical surgery was not the best routine treatment for breast cancer, came from the National Surgical Adjuvant Breast Project (NSABP) under the direction of Bernard Fisher, professor of surgery at the University of Pittsburgh. The group was started in 1957 when health specialists at the National Cancer Institute realized the virtual impossibility of answering important treatment questions by considering conflicting data from earlier studies. It was apparent that a researcher who spent enough time in a good medical library could build a strong case for just about any opinion by selectively choosing studies to support a favored view. To avoid such bias, the NSABP began a policy of pooling information from numerous hospitals and institutions that had agreed to assign informed volunteers randomly into different treatment programs. It was much like the British system.

When the consensus group met they knew that a NSABP study involving thirty-four institutions and some 1,700 women in the United States and Canada had recently found no difference in survival rates between women who had the radical mastectomy and those who had the less deforming total mastectomy.

The consensus meeting shattered ninety years of tradition. Three current studies—two in the United States and one in Italy—which are carefully surveying women randomly assorted into groups receiving either traditional surgery or breast-saving treatments could soon result in more drastic changes.

In July 1981, Italy's National Cancer Institute reported in the *New England Journal of Medicine* that it could find no difference in survival rates between women who received the radical mastectomy and those who, after having had a quarter of their breasts removed, received radiation. Seven hundred women whose tumors were less than an inch in diameter and whose lymph nodes appeared to be free of cancer participated in the project. Up to seven and a half years after surgery, there was no difference in either cancer recurrence or survival between the two groups. Eighty-three percent of those who had radical surgery and 84 percent of those with a partial mastectomy were alive and free of disease. Complications in treatment occurred in sixteen of 352 patients with limited surgery and radiation therapy and in twenty-three of 349 women treated by radical mastectomy.

Umberto Veronesi started the study in 1973. When he presented the findings at a recent national conference in the United States, he said it had been difficult to get Italian physicians to recommend that women volunteer for the study. "When we first started, they didn't like their patients getting the still unproven breast-saving surgery. A few years later they were reluctant because they didn't want women to receive the radical mastectomy." Unfortunately, once a study is under way, established treatment categories must be maintained to achieve meaningful results.

Findings are not yet in from similar studies started by the NSABP in 1976 and the National Cancer Institute in 1979. In the NSABP study, women are being put at random into one of three treatment groups. The first group undergoes a wedge resection or a large lumpectomy in which the lump and surrounding margin of tissue are removed. A second group receives the same treatment, followed by radiation therapy. A third group is treated by mastectomy.

Results will answer several important questions guaranteed to stir passionate debates at any medical conference. The first is, Does the woman who receives limited surgery really need radiation? The second deals with the controversial question of multicentric cancers, small microscopic cancers found in other parts of the breast as often as 50 percent of the time. Many doctors refuse to do limited surgery because they feel these growths may continue to develop and threaten a woman's life. Others disagree, contending that these microscopic cancers rarely develop into harmful invasive disease.

On this point, George Crile says, "We warn all our patients that if they want to conserve the breast they can do so without diminishing their chances of survival, but that there is a 20 percent chance of their having to have additional treatment. A partial mastectomy, therefore, can be considered as the first stage of what may be a two-stage operation. However, 80 percent of the patients never require the second stage and only 7.5 percent lose a breast."

At first glance, these studies are simply evaluating different kinds of treatment. But that only touches the surface of the problem. A deeper look shows that the tests are aimed at a revolutionary investigation of cancer growth and spread. The studies are really pitting old Halstedian theories against concepts that, if accepted, will make today's treatment, even with its new options, as obsolete as yesterday's radical surgery.

The old theory held that cancer grows in an orderly, predictable pattern, starting in one area of the breast. Upon reaching a certain size or stage, it spreads through the lymphatic vessels to the neighboring lymph nodes under the armpit. According to this theory, the nodes entangle the cancer like a fishnet, preventing it from spreading elsewhere, at least for a while. This concept led to the long-held belief that the extent of the operation affected a woman's chance of survival. The hope was that one more lymph node removed could save the patient's life.

Today, there is a new biology of cancer, whose chief defender is Bernard Fisher, chairman of the National Surgical Adjuvant Breast Project. This alternative theory, backed by laboratory and patient studies, contends that most, if not all, women who enter a doctor's office with a solid breast cancer have widely disseminated disease. Rather than being localized, cancer is a systemic disease that begins to shed cells into the bloodstream shortly after its birth. The theory also holds that cancer doesn't spread in an orderly, predictable fashion, and, in fact, from early on passes quite easily through the lymph nodes. Whether the nodes are negative or positive depends largely on how well the woman responds to the cancer attack. If the nodes are negative, (cancer-free) her immune system has done a good job of fighting the cancer and the rest of her body will put up a defense. Positive nodes (cancer is present) indicate that the cancer has escaped the body's natural defense system and is highly likely to thrive elsewhere. But some critics of this theory argue that cancer grows in a predictable and self-contained pattern, at least during its early development.

The theory forms the basis for using chemotherapy in a radically new way. When I had my surgery, it was a bad sign to be receiving chemotherapy, a sure indication that nothing else had worked and that cancer was overtaking the rest of the body. Now anticancer drugs are given routinely to a woman when cancer is detected in any of the lymph nodes under her arm. Drug treatment given before the disease shows up elsewhere is called "adjuvant chemotherapy." Studies have shown that even though these women don't have detectable signs of cancer in other parts of their bodies, the disease will reappear in 40 to 60 percent of them within five years' time. The decision to give chemotherapy to these high-risk but still healthy women was backed by animal studies that found the smaller the number of cells, the more effective the cancer drug. Cancer, when it reappears, contains as many as one billion cells, a difficult target to control.

Studies in the early 1970s by the National Cancer Institute found that small doses of one drug called L-Pam did delay recurrence in young women, but the protection wasn't as effective for older women. However, Betty Ford was one of the women who took the drug and encouraged others to try it.

In 1976, a major study from the National Cancer Institute of Milan reported findings that a three-drug combination was superior. Sixty-four percent of young (premenopausal) women who received the drugs were still cancer-free at the end of five years compared to 43 percent of women who were not treated with the three-drug combination. Results again were not as dramatic for older women.

Since the study came out, young women with positive nodes have been routinely placed on chemotherapy. Twenty-eight-year-old Sheila Jackson of Oakland is one who received a full year of adjuvant chemotherapy. Residents of California may have seen Sheila, in her graduation cap and gown, smiling from an American Cancer Society poster. The caption reads, "Last year Sheila had breast cancer. This year, she'll get her MBA" (Master of Business Administration).

Jackson was put on chemotherapy because two of the nineteen lymph nodes removed during her mastectomy were positive for cancer.

Twice a month for a year, she took a combination of drugs that left her jittery and exhausted for days. Yet she maintained a B average at Golden Gate University and was graduated only one semester behind schedule. It wasn't easy, but Jackson said she would probably do it again.

Statistics now show the first national downturn in death rates among young women. Between 1970 and 1978, death rates for older women went up about 1 percent per year, but rates for women under forty-five years of age dropped by 2 percent a year. (See the following figure.) Is the trend related to chemotherapy, and are these indications that many of these women are cured of their disease? We will know the answer to these questions in another 10 to 15 years.

World experts like Umberto Veronesi say chemotherapy shows promise of reducing death rates by 15 to 20 percent in high-risk patients. Bernard Fisher has predicted that adjuvant therapy will produce a major decline in death for all women in the next decade.

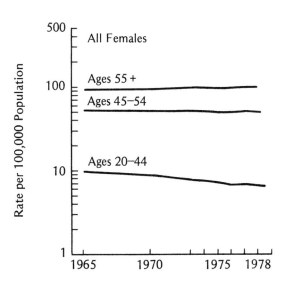

Breast Cancer Mortality Rates
in the United States
from 1965 to 1978

However, these are only predictions. For now, I agree with the San Francisco oncologist who said, "It's a difficult time to be a cancer patient. Patients want to know something definite, but the answers aren't available. It's difficult to accept, but data in this field are constantly changing."

The coming years are bound to see continuing investigation into new drug combinations and sequence of delivery. Today, as many as five drugs may be combined, and some researchers say they receive best results with mixtures of chemicals and hormones.

Another important question is, Will the drugs themselves produce long-term side effects? So far, no problems have been reported, but it will take time and the treatment of many thousands of women before a trend becomes obvious.

Uncertainty is the main reason adjuvant chemotherapy isn't being routinely given to women whose lymph nodes are negative. Fifteen percent of them will have problems within five years, and 25 percent will have problems within ten years. But is it wise to overtreat the 75 to 85 percent of women in this group who will be free of disease? The answer now is no, but studies are under way to spot the women most likely to have recurrence and to determine if the group as a whole benefits from adjuvant chemotherapy. Results could lead to new policies.

Adjuvant chemotherapy is only one example of how quickly treatments are changing. When I first started writing this book, studies showed that the drugs helped only women under fifty. Many centers and hospitals did not recommend it for postmenopausal breast cancer patients.

In January 1981, Milan's National Cancer Institute reported that older women didn't do as well because they hadn't received as much chemotherapy. Doctors cut back the doses, fearing full strength would be too toxic. But of those older women who received the stronger doses, 75 percent were disease-free at the end of five years compared to 49 percent of older women who didn't get treatment. Results were almost equal to those of younger women (77 percent versus 45 percent).

It's difficult for even the experts to keep up to date on such rapidly changing information. Until answers from controlled studies do come in, a woman's treatment is likely to be based on her doctor's training and beliefs, the amount of reading he or she has done, and the number of meetings he or she has attended.

Four women I've talked to recently typify how diverse options are and show how far we have come since the early 1970s, when most women were processed through one operation and treated by one doctor.

Brenda Winston, thirty-four, a grade-school teacher in Oakland, said her doctor discovered her lump during her annual physical examination. Her breasts are small, and the hard pea-sized lump was easy to detect. Outpatient biopsy showed that the lump was cancerous. Two surgeons advised her to have a modified radical mastectomy. She decided it was important for her to keep her breast so she also saw a radiation therapist who said she would be a good candidate for radiation therapy. Some lymph nodes were removed to determine if she needed chemotherapy. She didn't. Winston was treated three years ago and is fine today.

Kaye A. Heinz, a practical nurse from Virginia Beach, Virginia, was thirty-one in April 1977 when she discovered a hard lump in her breast. She had had fibrocystic disease for years, however, and didn't have the lump biopsied for several months. When she did, her surgeon found two types of cancer, including one (invasive lobular carcinoma) that has a high frequency of occurring in the second breast. Fortunately, no nodes were involved. Heinz decided to have both her breasts removed—"I didn't want to live with the fact that cancer could grow in my second breast"—and immediate reconstruction. She recalls, "I was actually excited about the operation. It might sound strange, but I couldn't wait to get on the operating table. I got rid of my cancer, and reconstruction gave me something to look forward to." Although the results do not match her former breasts, she is so happy with the results that she founded AWEAR (A Woman Educating About Reconstruction) in Virginia to help other women learn about reconstruction.

Betty, forty-five, is an extremely attractive woman who had a modified radical mastectomy five years ago. Three lymph nodes were positive, and she was immediately put on a year of chemotherapy. There have been no problems. Betty knows about reconstruction, but says she really isn't interested. "I just don't like the thought of something unnatural under my skin. I seem to have a difficult time adjusting to artificial products. I couldn't even wear contact lenses. But, most important, I had excellent surgery and can wear anything I want. I'm very happy just the way I am. I just want to keep on doing as much living as possible."

Sixty-two-year-old Jean Born, a recently retired education specialist who lives in San Francisco, posed a complicated problem as a woman who fit into the 5 percent group of patients who have cancer in both breasts. She had large breasts, her tumors were both very small, and her lymph nodes were negative. She wanted to keep her breasts and opted for radiation therapy, but there was concern about the consequences if tissue located between her breasts received double doses of radiation. She took her doctor's advice to have radiation therapy on one breast and a mastectomy and reconstruction on the other. She has finished her radiation treatments and set a date for reconstruction, still feeling well enough to continue swimming a mile several times a week.

The treatments were different and so were the women receiving them. Today, it's impossible to go back to the time the family doctor, relying solely on his own training and experience, decided what was best. Judgments are now based on what has happened to hundreds, if not thousands of women who have been checked for five, ten, and even twenty years.

The 1981 National Conference on Breast Cancer in San Diego offered an excellent chance to learn from many of the professionals involved in helping cancer patients. Pathologists, plastic surgeons, epidemiologists, oncologists, radiologists, radiation therapists, psychologists, genetic counselors, surgeons, and nurses all participated in a new team approach to treating breast cancer patients.

After a few days of hearing papers presented on a variety of topics, Donald Henson, chief of diagnostic procedures for the National Cancer Institute's Breast Cancer Task Force, said, "What you're really listening to is people politely disagreeing and defending their own specialties and turfs. But out of the differing opinions and shared information, the patient will benefit."

One of the newest members of this team is an oncologist, or cancer specialist. Before 1973, and at the time I had my surgery, oncology wasn't even a recognized specialty. Today, it is one of the fastest-growing specialties in medicine, second only to cardiology in the number of doctors who enter training programs each year. An oncologist is a good person to consult to review all treatment options because he or she can be more objective than, say, a surgeon or a radiologist, who is likely to be biased in favor of his or her particular specialty.

Social scientists also are a part of the cancer research team and are beginning to raise totally new questions and concerns about how women cope with their disease. Does it affect their marital or sexual life? Has it caused any family problems? Would they benefit from a support group? Has reconstruction been suggested? Quality of life is a growing new issue that is discussed increasingly at medical conferences, at which only new developments in surgery were formerly considered.

A major change of the last ten years is that more women want to participate in the decision-making process. With so many unknowns and no guarantees, no matter which treatment they follow, women say it's only fair that their priorities be heard. The changes are affecting the entire doctor-patient relationship.

It's hard to believe, but as recently as 1960 the majority of doctors preferred not to tell a patient that she had cancer. Breasts often were removed "because something looks suspicious" or because "something might develop into cancer." The most recent study in 1977 found that the vast majority of doctors tell the patients the truth. Today, many women say that they want to have still more information. Many want to know all their options as well as the risks and benefits of different procedures, so they can choose the treatment they prefer.

Shirley Temple Black investigated her options before deciding on treatment. "I have always taken the position that what happens to me should be, as far as is humanly possible, my own decision. Coming up with cancer would certainly not be my decision. But if it were cancer, what to do about it certainly would be." Black, who decided on a simple mastectomy and having a few lymph nodes removed, said she told herself, "My doctor can make the incision, but I want to make the decision."

In 1974, when journalist and science writer Rose Kushner discovered that the tiny bulge on the edge of her left nipple was cancer, she went to the nearest medical library to research her options and decided on the modified radical mastectomy. When she was denied the procedure at the National Cancer Institute, she flew to New York's Memorial Sloan-Kettering Cancer Center to consult a top breast cancer specialist. When she couldn't get a modified mastectomy there, she went to Roswell Park Memorial Institute in Buffalo, New York, where she found she was a good candidate for the procedure. The experience altered her life and turned her into a leading crusader for better health care for breast cancer patients.

Breast cancer itself has come out of the closet. Ten years ago many women felt embarrassed or ashamed to admit that they had a disease like breast cancer, which evoked all the negative images of cancer as well as feelings in some women that it could destroy their sexuality and femininity. In the 1970s, Betty Ford, Happy Rockefeller, Marvella Bayh, Shirley Temple Black, Julia Child, and Betty Rollin shared their own experiences with the disease. Although the messages weren't always optimistic, they helped women understand that there is no reason for secrecy and that a rewarding and fulfilling life can follow a diagnosis of breast cancer.

The concept of the second opinion is fairly new. When I first discovered my lump back in 1972, I wouldn't have dreamed of asking for a second opinion. It would have seemed too much of an insult to the doctor. I have matured considerably and seen how varied the results of treatment can be. Today I consider it an insult to myself not to try to get the best treatment and the most up-to-date information.

I'll never regret having sought second and third opinions when one plastic surgeon suggested that I might be a good candidate for reconstruction by a complicated microsurgical procedure. When I investigated, I learned that the procedure had a high (20 percent) complication rate and could have disastrous consequences. I saw the good results on one woman. However, I also heard that the procedure did not work on the plastic surgeon's next two patients. I still wonder what might have happened to me if I hadn't taken the time and spent the extra money for other opinions. When I learned the risks and the benefits, I could see that, for me, the risk was too great. It seemed a wise idea to at least give the procedure another year of use before volunteering to be a candidate. During that time, another procedure was developed that was more reliable, safer, and easier to go through. I was fortunate in being able to make a choice about elective surgery. I had time.

But getting a second opinion before you have an operation or start a recommended treatment doesn't have to take more than a few weeks. Another example of how valuable it can be was shown to me when I interviewed oncologists in different areas of the San Francisco Bay Area. One hospital regularly was giving chemotherapy to older women. Another was not using it routinely for older patients, obviously unaware of or unconvinced by new studies that reported survival rates were improved for older women when they received adequate doses.

Marion Morra and Eve Potts explain in *Choices*, "If at all possible, a second opinion is an absolute must at the start before submitting to any cancer treatment of any kind. This is not to suggest that the diagnosis you were given is not correct or that the suggested treatment might not be the best. It is only to say that you deserve the right to have the doctor's diagnosis reconfirmed and alternative treatments explored and explained to you."

Vincent DeVita, director of the National Cancer Institute, said in an April 15, 1981, *New York Times* interview, "When you face any disease that may kill you, don't rely on the judgment of a single person. A second opinion is especially important if the first doctor has a pessimistic view of your chances of recovery."

I think that consumerism and the women's movement, which is making it easier for women to get information, are helping to spotlight many problems in health care today, especially those surrounding breast cancer.

I was fortunate to learn about Images and Options, a San Francisco area group that provides information on reconstruction, when I needed help in making an intelligent decision. Other groups provide similar services in other parts of the country: RENU (Reconstruction Education for National Understanding) in Washington, D.C., and the Cleveland area; AFTER (Ask a Friend to Explain Reconstruction) in New York; and AWEAR (A Woman Educating About Reconstruction) in the Richmond, Virginia, area. Their numbers are listed in Appendix G.

Volunteers provide information over the telephone, help put you in contact with someone who has already had reconstruction, and may hold group meetings—all aimed at helping you make informed decisions.

Rose Kushner, after helping to champion the case against the radical mastectomy, has started a Breast Cancer Advisory Center in Maryland. The group sends out free fact sheets on breast care problems. The address is in Appendix G.

When all else has failed, women have been influential in getting state laws passed to protect their rights. In May 1979, Massachusetts passed a Patient's Rights Bill requiring that a patient suffering from any form of breast cancer be given complete information on all medically viable alternative treatments. In September 1980, California enacted a law requiring physicians to give breast cancer patients a written summary of medically viable alternative methods of treatment. The statement was developed by the state's Cancer Advisory Council. Both Marjorie Roach, who worked to get the Massachusetts Bill passed, and Juliet Ristom, who championed the California law, said that their doctors had tried to railroad them into having mastectomies.

Marjorie Roach recalls that when she asked about radiation therapy her doctor replied, "How many children do you have? How old are they? Don't you think that they need you? I have heard others talk like you ..." "This man had left me death as the only alternative," said Roach.

We have entered the 1980s with more change than ever before; the constants that virtually every one agrees on are that some treatment is better than no treatment and that the woman who discovers her lump early has the best chance for long-term survival. Removing the tumor, by whichever procedure, at least stops the shedding of cells and makes it easier for the body to defend itself.

Early detection also means you are much more likely to get the best results from new options like radiation therapy and reconstruction. If you have a small tumor the doctors won't have to remove as much tissue in the biopsy, and your remaining breast will be more natural if you choose radiation. And if the tumor is small, the surgeon can leave more skin during a mastectomy. You should get better results from reconstruction, certainly avoiding the more complicated procedures that provide additional skin.

The most important reason for finding a tumor early, however, is that the smaller the tumor, the lower the risk that lymph nodes are involved. According to today's two competing explanations, either your immune system has been able to keep cancer cells under control or, alternately, cancer cells simply have not started to spread.

Whichever condition applies, if cancer is discovered and treated before it spreads to the lymph nodes, you have an 85 percent chance of living five years and close to a 75 percent chance of living ten years.

(See the accompanying figure.) Some women in the latter group, having been cured, can live a normal life—at least long enough to die from another cause.

When nodes are involved, the five-year survival rate drops to 56 percent and the ten-year survival rate to about 40 percent. How chemotherapy will affect these figures is still uncertain, but even if it does significantly improve life expectancy, it also exposes you to side effects and the possibility of future unknown problems, risks worth taking in my view, but still unnecessary if a lump is found early.

The real tragedy in breast cancer is that it is the leading cause of cancer deaths in women and the leading cause of all deaths among

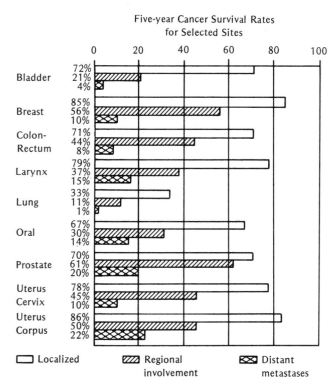

Five-year Cancer Survival Rates for Selected Sites

Source: Biometry Branch, National Cancer Institute. Courtesy American Cancer Society.

women forty to forty-four years old. Statistics show that until recently, mortality rates from breast cancer had not changed in fifty years. By the time half the women show up in a doctor's office with a lump, their disease has spread. Most women still find the lumps themselves, when the average size is well over an inch in diameter. An American College of Surgeons report found that cancer is contained in the breast area in 50 percent of such cases; it is involved in the lymph nodes in 40 percent of cases and has already become involved in other areas of the body in 7 percent of cases.

The only way to change these figures is through early detection, which is best achieved through routine breast self-examination and an occasional low-dose mammogram. A 1980 report from the National Cancer Institute found that almost every woman has heard of breast self-examination, but only 40 percent used the technique monthly or more frequently. And although 61 percent of women had heard of mammography, only 19 percent reported having had a mammogram.

The most important choice women have today may be in giving themselves the best chance against breast cancer by knowing the value of early detection. Until recently a woman's reward for finding a lump was having her breast removed. Today, women no longer have to pay that price.

Some see today's unanswered questions and change as confusing and a time for pessimism. I think we are fortunate to have progressed into a new age when the "experts" are publicly admitting their limitations, recognizing that they don't have complete answers. Finally, cancer specialists are asking the right and the more humane questions.

CHAPTER 6

It's Cancer—Now What Happens?

If your diagnosis comes in as cancer, the most important point to remember is that you have not just been handed a death sentence. I don't say that to diminish the threat of breast cancer. I have known women who have died of the disease.

But I am a realist and working as a Reach to Recovery volunteer has helped me meet many others who are true inspirations. These volunteers are alive, well, leading full, productive lives ten, fifteen, and even twenty years after learning that they had breast cancer.

Sixty-five-year-old Rachel Gillespie, a physical education teacher in a Hayward, California, high school is one of the many women I look forward to seeing each year at the Reach to Recovery training sessions. "I had my surgery nineteen years ago," she recalls. "There have been a lot of changes and improvements in treatments since I left the hospital with a sanitary napkin in my bra for a breast form. Back then there was no visit from a Reach to Recovery volunteer, and little chance to talk to anybody else who had had the disease, which I think is important. Women seemed especially leery of talking about breast cancer. It was almost as though they thought it was contagious."

Gillespie says her only problem now, when she has a minor ailment, is convincing doctors that it isn't cancer. In addition to teaching full time, through the Reach to Recovery program she visits women in the hospital who have had a mastectomy and does volunteer work at a hospital information desk. She gets plenty of exercise through teaching—volleyball, basketball, baseball—and enjoys swimming, bowling, and tennis when not working. She has painted the outside of her house twice in the last ten years. Nobody would call her a cancer patient. She lost that epithet years ago.

When I found that I had cancer, there were certainly times I expected the worst. Like many people, I became a victim of the myths surrounding cancer and ignored the facts that show how many people live after having the disease. When my cold forced me to delay my biopsy, I visited the company nurse a few times each day to drink an aspirin-and-vitamin concoction that helped my sore throat and kept my temperature down. I noticed that the man who sat two desks away from me, an energetic and talented thirty-year-old new addition to the staff, was visiting the nurse as often as I was. He said he was taking something for a bleeding ulcer. I suspect that if we both had known we soon would be having surgery, given the choice of our disease each of us would have preferred to be treated for the ulcer.

Shortly after I returned to work, the young man died from an infection that developed after the ulcer operation. I was shocked. How could he die from an ulcer and how could I who had cancer be told that I had an excellent chance of being cured and living a long life? If I could live for five more years, to reach his age, I would be happy. Five years passed, and soon it will be ten years since my operation. What can I say, but that cancer, especially if caught early, is not another name for death.

Some women equate the disease with death because they have known others who have died of breast cancer. This isn't a good comparison. Your neighbor's or aunt's experience with breast cancer isn't likely to happen to you because breast cancer isn't one disease, but as many as fifteen different diseases. Each carries its individual characteristics and prognosis. Some breast cancers are more likely to spread than others. One type grows rapidly; others are very lazy. Most breast tumors grow at a slower pace than other types of cancer.

And just as breast cancers vary in their growth patterns, so do women vary in their responses to treatment. Some women have a stronger defense against cancer than others. Older women respond differently to treatment than younger ones. The number of lymph nodes involved, whether none, one to three, or four or more is another variable. The course of your disease is affected by whether your tumor is under the influence of your body's natural hormone levels, i.e., whether it is estrogen positive or estrogen negative.

If you have this information, you can begin to understand your treatment options and make the best choices with your doctor. It will probably be difficult to make decisions after being confronted with the diagnosis of cancer. That's one good reason to be at least minimally informed about this common problem before you have to deal with it. The odds are that you won't have to go through the experience. But I'm convinced that being informed and knowing the right questions to ask and where to go for help can help reduce the panic and fear that a cancer diagnosis can bring. One woman said, "I can go through just about anything if I know what is happening. Women go through the pain of childbirth by learning how to breathe correctly. Certainly the treatments for breast cancer can't be more difficult."

You may feel that doing nothing and refusing to make any decision is a tempting option. It's a choice, and some women who have refused all treatments have lived as long as twenty years. The average life expectancy, however, is only two and a half years. One doctor called this choice, "a slow and painful form of suicide."

Even when you're trying to concentrate and make decisions, you may have a problem understanding new medical terms, all the options, and how they apply to you, which is a normal reaction. One physician explained, "Patients seem to remember very little of what doctors tell them, particularly when anxiety or denial prevail; they tend to focus on key words or phrases and blot out the rest."

Ernest H. Rosenbaum, a San Francisco cancer specialist, relates such a reaction: "After consultation with a patient, her mother, and sister, including a forty-minute discussion on future tests, treatments, and a detailed explanation of radiation therapy and chemotherapy, I walked the patient to the door of my office. Her cousin met her at the door and asked, 'What did the doctor tell you?' She answered, 'I forgot.' "

However, he has devised ways to deal with the problem. Since 1975 Rosenbaum has tape-recorded his initial diagnostic discussion with each individual patient. He gives the tape cassette to the patient and if necessary also loans a recorder.

"I hope the recorded information heard in a private, calmer, more rational moment, will help the patient understand available medical treatment and give her realistic hope for the future," he said. Another advantage is that future visits can be used to build on information and understanding rather than just repeating and reviewing the first visit.

Rosenbaum and other patient advocates suggest that a family member or friend be present during the early discussion sessions with your doctor. They should be encouraged to ask questions. Being able to discuss your choices with somebody else may help clarify what is important to you. It can help identify the problems and fears you have to work out with your doctor.

Brenda Winston believes, "It is critical that a woman be able to go through the experience with a good friend, husband, relative, someone who is willing to become informed and participate in discussions with your doctor. At times, I just stopped listening or got so choked up that I couldn't listen. Having my husband there to help reexplain things and to repeat what was really said helped. Don't go through it alone, no matter what."

During less traumatic times than your first appointment, you may find communication easier if you write all your questions down on a piece of paper before you enter a doctor's office for your appointment. And don't feel foolish about taking a notebook so you can jot down responses. It's also smart to ask for definitions when you are unsure what new words mean.

A good question to ask yourself early in treatment is whether your doctor seems committed to working with you and is well qualified to treat cancer patients. Does the doctor treat a lot of cancer patients? For example, the average general surgeon sees about ten breast cancer patients a year; specialists average about ten patients a week.

Another question: Do you want to be treated at a Comprehensive Cancer Center or a teaching hospital? Qualified cancer specialists in community hospitals can provide you with very good standard procedures and treatments. However, you're likely to get the most up-to-date care in cancer centers or teaching hospitals. The twenty-one Comprehensive Cancer Centers listed in Appendix F have been designated by the National Cancer Institute as "institutes of excellence" for treating cancer patients. The centers conduct a broad range of research and are dedicated to finding better methods of cancer prevention, diagnosis, treatment, and rehabilitation.

The only negative comment I have heard about the cancer centers came from Cleveland surgeon George Crile, who cautioned that you're most likely to find doctors committed to the radical mastectomy in such centers. Even in the Bay Area, although some doctors at one medical center are routinely offering lumpectomies or modified radicals, their colleague, a doctor at the same center, still almost routinely does the radical mastectomy. What it comes down to is that even at teaching hospitals and cancer centers, you still have to assume some burden of responsibility for your own care.

Breast cancer is one area in which promising new treatments are being investigated, and you should ask yourself if you want to participate in a clinical study. Although many women think they are being guinea pigs, investigative programs have excellent track records for comparing the best standard treatment in use against a possibly more promising experimental treatment. In most cases, patients in experimental programs do better than women receiving more traditional treatment.

Vincent DeVita, director of the National Cancer Institute, said that although many issues are debated today, the fact that women get the best treatment in clinical studies is not one of them. Rigid record keeping, close supervision, and psychological and support services are readily available. Benefits and risks are clearly outlined for women before they enter the studies.

As of April 1980, more than 150 clinical trials on breast cancer were under way in the United States. Most are testing new drug combinations. One is considering ways for women to control stress while undergoing chemotherapy, and some studies, already mentioned in Chapter 5, are evaluating new types of surgery and radiation therapy.

The reasons for entering clincial study programs vary. Allen S. Lichter, head of radiation therapy at the National Cancer Institute, said women tell him they participate in the Institute's trials because some feel they are getting better care, especially if they live in medically underserved areas. Others say they get a more balanced perspective and that it's better than just getting advice from one doctor. Some tell him that they want to make their case count and contribute toward increased knowledge. Finally, some are poor and can't afford medical care; they volunteer because some studies pay all medical costs, including transportation if required.

Most clinical studies are conducted at Comprehensive Cancer Centers and teaching centers, but you may volunteer at a community hospital if your doctor is a participant. If you are interested, discuss it with your oncologist or call one of the National Cancer Institute's toll-free information numbers listed in Appendix E. The free telephone service was started in 1979 to answer the public's questions about cancer and to provide information about studies for which you may be eligible.

Knowing if your disease is already located in your lymph nodes or in other areas of your body may help you decide whether you would gain by participating in an ongoing study or traveling to a cancer center for care or review of your case. Answers about the extent of disease are accumulated for every cancer patient by a process called "staging." The information helps doctors communicate with each other about your specific case and compile records on what happens to women who share similar disease characteristics.

Classification into one of four stages is determined by the results of several medical tests plus the surgeon's observations when he or she removed your tumor during biopsy and the pathologist's examination under the microscope of your tumor and lymph nodes. Your particular stage assignment tells a lot about your prognosis and treatment options.

Stage I involves a small tumor (smaller than one inch in diameter), no lymph node spread, and no spread to other organs. Your disease is considered limited to your breast and your prognosis is excellent.

Stage II consists of a tumor between one and two inches across (2 to 5 cm). You may have some lymph nodes involved with your cancer, but there is no evidence of spread. You are still considered to have early breast cancer, and a good prognosis, but you will be recommended for adjuvant chemotherapy if any lymph nodes show the presence of cancer cells.

Remember, cancer contained in a breast won't kill anybody. Your life is seriously threatened only when the cancer cells leave your breast and invade, take over, and eventually destroy more critical organs like the liver and lungs.

A Stage III tumor is larger than two inches. Lymph nodes are almost always involved with cancer cells, often at an advanced stage where the malignant cells also are invading other surrounding tissue and causing the nodes to become fixed to each other. However, there is still no sign of spread to more distant organs.

In Stage IV tests picked up evidence of spread of cancer cells to other areas of your body, most likely the liver, bones, lungs, or brain.

Women with early breast cancer will be excellent candidates for the total mastectomy with axillary dissection. A good plastic surgeon can perform reconstruction, usually with good results. More and more doctors are offering women with early breast cancer a lumpectomy followed by radiation treatments.

For Stage III tumors, which are large and bulky, most doctors suggest a mastectomy, possibly with follow-up reconstruction. However, large-breasted women with Stage III cancers may be considered for lumpectomy and radiation.

With advanced cancer (Stage IV) all efforts should be aimed at controlling the disease and prolonging survival. In fact, there should be no reason to do a mastectomy except to make the patient more comfortable—if, for example, the tumor is causing pain or threatening to ulcerate.

Shirley Temple Black took this into consideration when she made her choice. In an article on her life that appeared in *Good Housekeeping* in February 1981 she said she decided to have a mastectomy because studies had shown that her cancer had not spread. "I think if the cancer had spread all over my body (which it hadn't), maybe I would have chosen not to have any surgery at all." There would have been no reason. She said she would have preferred to keep her breast and live "as long as I was supposed to."

But women are still having their breasts removed today and then learning that they have advanced cancer, a sign that they weren't properly evaluated and tested before the operation.

The common work-up tests critical for determining if your disease has spread are a mammogram on your opposite breast, a chest x-ray and blood and urine studies. A mammogram is requested because with cancer in one breast there is about a 5 percent chance of cancer in your second breast. The mammogram also can be used as a baseline record against which doctors can measure future breast changes. Chest x-rays determine if cancer has spread to your lungs or ribs, and blood studies can provide early information of liver and bone involvement.

Some doctors may also suggest liver and bone scans. They sound awful, but are really quite painless. Both work on the same principle—that weak radioactive substances injected into your bloodstream will collect in different amounts in normal cells and in cancerous cells. In the liver, cancerous cells do not show as much of the substance as normal cells. It's just the opposite in the bones. Once the material is injected into your body, you will have to wait a few hours for it to accumulate in amounts large enough so that a special camera going over your body can scan and record the distribution of the substance.

Doctors actively involved in research are more likely to ask for liver and bone scans than are practicing community physicians. The reason is that the tests are expensive and results are questionable or show up at about the same time as obvious liver distress or bone pain. For example, the liver scan rarely finds cancers under an inch in diameter. The bone scan, in contrast, is so sensitive that it often picks up old fractures, injuries, arthritis, and infection.

I had the series of tests at the time of my mastectomy and again at the request of my plastic surgeon before reconstruction five years later. I didn't object to the tests after my mastectomy, although it certainly would have made more sense to have a work-up before my operation than after, a procedure more commonly done today. I did question the necessity and value of having the expensive (over $500) and time-consuming battery of tests repeated before my reconstruction. I didn't like the extra exposure to radiation, besides, I felt I was in excellent health. In fact, I can remember taking my jogging clothes with me on the day of one of my tests and jogging more than a mile through San Francisco's Golden Gate Park while waiting for the radioactive substance to settle in my liver so I could be scanned.

I remember musing, "This is absurd. If somebody I know comes up and asks why I'm jogging through the park this morning instead of working . . . I could imagine their shock if I explained that I was being scanned for cancer."

Still, I felt good afterward, knowing I had a clean bill of health again. However, what I know now about the overall accuracy of the tests makes me question even more why I needed them. If anything, they gave me a false sense of reassurance. If I had understood their value, I could have had an intelligent conversation with my plastic surgeon over why he requested the scans. The problem, of course, was that I simply didn't know the right questions to ask then. "Why do I need this test?" "How accurate is it?" are two questions I'm learning to ask more often.

There is good news about cancer diagnosis. Largely as a result of mammography, an entirely new category of highly curable cancers, called "minimal," is being discovered. Some cancers grouped in this category are small—less that one half inch (1 cm) in diameter. They can't be felt by even the most experienced doctor or nurse. If invasion has started, it is usually confined to the breast.

Other cancers in this category are called "noninvasive" or "in situ," (literally meaning "in place"), because they are contained in the milk ducts in which they originated. The cancerous cells have not yet begun to spread into surrounding breast tissue, much less the lymph nodes or the body. Survival rates are excellent with these types of cancer—some say over 93 percent at twenty years.

Now the bad news. There is probably more disagreement over how to treat these minimal cancers than over any other type of breast cancer. Experts are poles apart on what should be done. Some say you should have only a lumpectomy and be closely followed. Others advise that since some types of minimal cancers often involve both breasts, you should have them both removed.

These cancers are more difficult to diagnose accurately than other types of cancers. In twenty-seven breast cancer screening centers mammography alone detected over 500 real minimal cancers, but it also spotted 48 benign growths that were misdiagnosed as cancer.* Thirty-seven women underwent needless mastectomies. The mistake came to light when other pathologists reviewed all cancers diagnosed as minimal in the screening program.

A 1977 Consensus Development Conference on Breast Cancer Screening recommended "concurrent pathological review" of all minimal cancers so that any danger of misinterpreting the diagnoses would be entirely eliminated. However, these conferences have no power to enforce their recommendations and it may fall to you to make certain your results have been reviewed by at least two pathologists.

Rosamond Campion learned that she had minimal breast cancer in 1971. She refused to go along with her surgeon's suggestion to have a one-step procedure during which he would do a radical mastectomy if the lump proved to be cancerous. "I was," she said, "the first woman he ever knew to refuse to sign a consent form. I was being very silly and stubborn. It was essential, he told me, for a woman to put unquestioning faith in her doctor. The doctor always knows best."

Campion had the two-step procedure, however, and her tumor turned out to be noninvasive and less than one third inch in diameter. Instead of submitting to the radical mastectomy that had been suggested, she found a doctor who would remove only a small segment

---

*The number originally was listed as sixty-six cases, but on "review of the review" sixteen were rediagnosed as cancer and two were credited to computer error.

of tissue that surrounded the area where her lump had appeared. Her decision generated a flurry of criticism, both from doctors and from women. She said that on one television panel, an old New England surgeon had admitted grudgingly, "You're a pioneer." "Pioneer nothing," snapped a woman who had undergone a radical mastectomy in the 1930s. "She's a guinea pig and she'll regret being unwise."

Five years later, Campion wrote that she had no regrets about her decision. But she said, "The choice I made was right for me. I did not, do not, cannot recommend it for every woman."

It should be noted that even the doctor who performed her surgery might have reacted quite differently if her cancer had begun to invade the surrounding breast tissue. At the very least, he probably would have suggested that her treatment be combined with radiation therapy. Some doctors today also would suggest that she have some lymph nodes removed or sampled to see if they contain cancer. Even small cancers sometimes involve lymph nodes. If they were cancerous, her doctor would suggest adjuvant chemotherapy.

Children's Hospital in San Francisco provides a choice of treatments for minimal cancer. Pathologist Michael D. Lagios said the new options aren't based on pathologists reading the slides any differently, but rather on how much weight they want to give to assuring the patient that she won't get cancer.

He explained, "In the past, doctors would say, 'We're going to make all the decisions for you. You won't have to think and we're going to guarantee you that you won't get breast cancer. That means we're going to take off both your breasts.' I look at it differently. The woman should have a role in deciding her treatment and should understand the risks. Some women who don't want to take any risk at all elect to have their breasts removed. Others prefer to be followed and this is fine too."

To make an intelligent decision, one should be aware that there are two very different types of "in situ" cancers—lobular and ductal. Both types develop from an excess of cells formed in your milk ducts; but they look very different under a microscope.

Ductal cancer "in situ" is the more aggressive of the two. Evidence suggests that even if a ductal-type tumor is removed, there is still as much as a 50 percent chance that another cancer will develop later in the same breast. On the average, it will appear within ten years of a biopsy. It also is estimated that 33 to 75 percent of women will have other microscopic cancerlike growths in other parts of the same breast.

Most doctors would recommend a mastectomy or perhaps a lumpectomy and radiation therapy for a ductal-type tumor. However, Lagios says studies suggest that small ductal cancers in situ—those under one inch in diameter—aren't as aggressive as larger ones or as likely to be accompanied by other cancers in the same breast. He is currently following a group of twenty-two women who had these small cancers and opted to have only a lumpectomy. Results look promising, but it is still too early to draw definite conclusions.

Lobular cancer in situ presents a totally different picture. It was only described in 1941 after being detected in three women who subsequently developed invasive breast cancer. The fact that these three women got breast cancer persuaded most doctors to recommend mastectomy as the best treatment when any woman was diagnosed with the problem.

Recent studies raise questions about routine mastectomy. One study reported that if you have a lobular in situ cancer removed, there is only an 11 percent chance that you'll ever develop a second breast cancer. Another study holds that the risk is closer to 30 percent. Both agree, however, that these subsequent cancers are sluggish and often take as long as twenty years to appear. More confusing, when they do appear, the odds are as great that they will appear in the opposite breast as in the one that contained the original cancer. Small multicentric cancers are also believed to be quite common in these breasts.

The evidence leads some doctors to suggest that both breasts be removed, but others believe that treatment is far too drastic. They say that 70 to 90 percent of women will never have a second cancer and a recurrence can appear in either breast. These doctors aren't as concerned about the significance of the multicentric lesions because no one can predict whether the cancerlike objects will ever progress to true cancers. As a result women are given a choice between having a mastectomy and being closely followed.

Minimal cancer is truly a bittersweet disease. Some women may consider you fortunate to have found a cancer with such a favorable prognosis. But I doubt they would envy the decision you have to make. The National Cancer Institute is currently evaluating the results of various therapies, but it is not ready to make any recommendations.

Experts at the 1981 National Conference on Breast Cancer were as divided as the medical profession in general on treatment options. Suggestions ranged from a biopsy and follow-up to prophylactic mastectomies of both breasts. However, this group agreed that they would be more likely to suggest routine follow-up as an option if the woman seemed willing to share the responsibility of her choice. That translates into routine and thorough self-examination, additional checkups at four- to six-month intervals from a doctor or a nurse, and periodic mammograms.

The majority of women who discover lumps today do not enjoy the excellent prognosis associated with minimal cancers. However, it is important to put the factors that affect a woman's prognosis into perspective before listing them.

The old pronouncements "He will be dead in six months" and "I will give him a year to live" are unforgivable statements for a physician to make, according to J. Englebert Dunphy, former head of surgery at the University of California at San Francisco, who over his long career has treated more cancer patients than most doctors.

"It's unforgivable," he says, "because there are not valid grounds to make so rigid a prognosis. It may be three months, six months, six years, or longer. One can never tell. One thing I have learned is that if a patient is told he is going to die in six months and doesn't, he never forgives the doctor." Dunphy says he doesn't try to present an unrealistic picture, but suggests odds and percentages, leaving ample room for shorter or longer periods of complete well-being.

The odds and percentages are definitely available, and your doctor shouldn't hide the information or minimize its importance. But, on the other hand, it would be a mistake to accept the results as the calendar your life will follow. The information is useful in helping to plan your life rather than to retreat into a shell and stop living it.

Ann, who lived in the San Francisco area and who wrote about her experience with cancer in *Decision for Life*, would have agreed completely with Dunphy. In December 1975—two years after her mastectomy—Ann was told that she had a year to live. Cancer had spread to her lung, then her hipbone and her liver. She had her ovaries removed in an effort to slow down the growth of the cancer and received radiation therapy to relieve the pain she felt in her hipbone. Instead of accepting the prognosis she decided to take control of her life, define her needs, and fill the rest of her time learning to live instead of learning to die.

One of her first steps was to find a doctor who did not take away all hope for cure. "I simply was not willing to work with a doctor who gave me no hope," she said. "My new doctor at least says he doesn't know what will happen to me. He is open to the possibility of life and not bent on playing God. He is concerned for me, my beliefs, values, and feelings."

In addition to her traditional medical treatment, Ann saw a psychiatrist, investigated meditation and relaxation exercises, improved her nutrition, and started to work on relationship difficulties with her husband. Two years later—spring 1977—she wrote, "I am feeling optimistic. I lead a normal life doing all the things a mother of five is required to do. I also attend classes in interior design, play tennis, and generally enjoy and appreciate my life. My consciousness has never been greater and there is room for further expansion."

Although I would like to be able to write that Ann had a complete remission and disappearance of her disease, the truth is that she died in March 1979. She had a bad prognosis and she knew it, but she also lived more than three years after hearing the ominous news that she had only one year left to live.

The single factor most predictive of ten- and twenty-year survival is the number of lymph nodes involved with your tumor. Although the prognosis worsens with each additional node found, women with four or more positive nodes have the worst prognosis.

Tumor size is important. For example, 80 percent of women with tumors less than one half inch in diameter, 55 percent of patients with tumors over one inch, and 45 percent of patients with tumors over two inches remain alive after ten years.

The type of tumor influences survival. The breast cancer that carries the very worst prognosis—inflammatory cancer—is fortunately rare, affecting fewer than 2 percent of all patients. The breast becomes reddened, thickened, tender to the touch, and looks infected. Average survival with this disease is less than two years.

Ductal cancer—the kind I had—is by far the most common type, accounting for nearly 80 percent of breast cancers in women. The following table, Tumor Type and Prognosis, lists six of the most common types of breast cancer, the average size of a woman's tumor when she

Tumor Type and Prognosis

Tumor Type:	Ductal	Lobular	Medullary	Colloid	Comedo	Papillary
Percentage of Total	78.1	8.7	4.3	2.6	4.6	1.2
Average Age [years]	51	54	49	50	49	52
Average Size [inches]	1.2	1.4	1.3	1.5	1.5	1.3
Node Involvement	60%	60%	44%	32%	32%	17%
Survival						
5 yrs.	59%	57%	69%	76%	84%	89%
10 yrs.	47%	42%	68%	72%	77%	65%
20 yrs.	38%	34%	62%	62%	74%	65%

Source: *Atlas of Tumor Pathology*, 2nd series, Washington D.C.: Armed Forces Institute of Pathology, 1967. Derived from twenty-year follow-up study of 1,458 patients with infiltrating breast cancer, all of whom were treated with radical mastectomy at the Memorial Hospital or James Ewing Hospital between 1940 and 1943.

Survival Rates Based on Lymph Node Status

	Recurrence			*Survival*	
	18 Months	*5 Years*	*10 Years*	*5 Years*	*10 Years*
No Nodes Involved	5%	18%	24%	78%	65%
Positive Nodes	33	65	76	46	25
1 to 3 Nodes	13	50	64	62	38
4 or More Nodes	52	79	86	32	13
All Patients	17	40	50	64	46

Source: Abstracted from data of the National Surgical Adjuvant Breast Program. B. Fisher et al, *Ann. Surg.* 168:337, 1968, and B. Fisher et al, *Surg. Gynecol. Obstet.* 140:528, 1975.

first visits a doctor, whether nodes are involved, and the resulting five-, ten-, and twenty-year survival rates.

Individual tumors may take from a few days to more than a year to double in size. Women with slow-growing tumors have a better prognosis than women with ones that grow rapidly.

Estrogen receptor status is the most recently discovered prognostic factor. The test is the same as that performed on tumors when they are first biopsied to help predict individual response to hormone manipulation should a cancer reappear. The test gives clues to if and when cancer will reappear. Women with an estrogen-positive tumor have an improved prognosis and generally will be free from disease longer than those with estrogen-negative tumors. Younger women and those going through menopause tend to have lower rates of estrogen-positive cancers than older women.

Again, these signs offer odds and predictions, but they leave room for many exceptions, both for better and worse. For example, 20 percent of women with relatively small tumors—those under one third of an inch in diameter—will have nodular involvement, possibly because they have extremely virulent types of cancer or their bodies do not have strong natural systems of defense. And more than one third of women with fairly large tumors—bigger than two inches—will be very fortunate to have no sign of spread.

Lucy Shapero learned to live with a poor prognosis and wrote about her experience in *Never Say Die*. On New Year's Eve 1969, she discovered a lump while taking a shower and preparing to go to a party. She started the first month of the year by learning the worst: the lump was cancerous. A radical mastectomy followed, and twenty-three out of thirty lymph nodes turned out to be cancer-positive.

She explained, "When I learned I had breast cancer, I was certain I was going to die. I was only thirty-seven years old, but I planned no further. For me, cancer was a single disease marked by terrible pain and a slow, torturous death. I was medically ignorant. I simply allowed what happened to happen. If I had admitted that the disease was a possibility in my life and had learned about the treatment procedures before I was diagnosed, I could have made the decisions that I live with today. But I didn't want to deal with the unpleasantness. The thought of breast cancer was so ugly. So why think of it."

In spite of the large number of lymph nodes involved, she lived for five years without any recurrence, already beating the odds. Then she found the disease had spread to a bone in her neck. "I knew I had no control of the cancer. I had accepted that. But I could have control over how I lived with that cancer. I could manage my life. I had prepared myself for death. Now I would learn how to live."

By the end of ten years, her children were grown, her husband well established in his work: "The way to live well with cancer is to want to live. To know that there are things I have to do. That I am needed. There is unknown joy on the threshold. To know that I can control my life—have controlled it—will control it. I have survived ten years. I want more." Lucy, like many women with breast cancer, had learned to face reality, and also to turn toward life. In September of 1981, she is still fine, completly free from any problems. "I know it has to do with my attitude," she said. "Both cancer patients and their doctors are too quick to accept that once cancer has spread, there isn't much hope left." She laughed, "The last time I saw my oncologist he said 'You'll probably live longer than I will.' "

Many would agree with Lucy that attitude is important in helping fight a disease. Today, women like Lucy who have lymph nodes involved with cancer have more reason for optimism because of adjuvant chemotherapy, the major new hope in the 1980s for treating healthy but high-risk breast cancer patients. Although there are still frustrating unknowns about chemotherapy, a woman can take some control of her treatment by selecting a cancer specialist who is knowledgeable and up to date on the best drugs to use

One thing is certain. Chemotherapy produces side effects, the most severe appearing the days you are taking the drugs. San Francisco oncologist Brian Lewis estimates that the majority of women given the drugs "function at least at 60 to 70 percent of their normal capacity. Five to 10 percent of patients have so much difficulty that they may decide to quit, and another 5 to 10 percent don't even know that they are taking therapy."

A mistake many women make when they are recommended for adjuvant chemotherapy is to compare their treatment and side effects to those of other women with advanced cancer or with other forms of cancer. A healthy woman should find it easier to tolerate treatments simply because she is healthy, well nourished, and able to recover faster than someone else who is fighting advanced disease.

Sheila Jackson has vivid memories of her year's treatment, a program that didn't stop her from continuing graduate studies. "Sometimes I would get so sick at night that I couldn't sleep. Now that I look back on it, I think I was doing quite well just to be well groomed, attractive, and pleasant." Jackson relied heavily on marijuana to help combat nausea. "It calmed my system and allowed my body to relax," she said, adding that it upsets her that politicians haven't legalized the drug for cancer patients. "I suggest that they take a few treatments. Then they will know why it is coldhearted to deny cancer patients relief."

Today's most commonly used drugs and their specific side effects are listed in Appendix D, but new information about alternative treatments appears monthly, so don't be surprised or worried if your drugs aren't listed. There are at least twenty different drugs to choose from and they work in different ways as cancer cells pass through routine cycles of growth, rest, and division. Always given in combination today, some drugs kill the cancer cell just as it is preparing to divide and double itself. Some aren't as picky and try to destroy the cell over its entire life. It's most difficult to kill the cell during its resting stage. So far efforts to lure the cancer cells out of their resting state have not been successful. In another tactic, a drug masquerades as normal nutrients and, in effect, starves the cell to death.

Although treatment combinations vary, all contain drugs that destroy the cancer cell as it is preparing to divide. Since not all cells divide at any one time only a certain percentage can be killed during any one cycle. That's why it's necessary to repeat the dose for maximum effectiveness. Today, you are most likely to receive drugs over a twelve-month cycle, although both shorter and longer cycles are under investigation.

Animal studies show that the time of starting treatment makes a difference in how effective response will be. This is one reason doctors may be reluctant to place a patient on chemotherapy later than three to six months after her lump is biopsied. Some doctors even question the wisdom of delaying chemotherapy while a woman who has had a lumpectomy completes five to seven weeks of radiation therapy. They prefer to give at least a few sessions of chemotherapy before starting radiation therapy. One oncologist said he doesn't like to give radiation and chemotherapy at the same time because side effects are intensified and more difficult for the patient to tolerate.

Side effects frequently develop from drugs that kill rapidly growing cells because the drugs aren't yet sophisticated enough to distinguish between cancer cells and normal cells. The result: rapidly growing normal cells are also sacrificed.

Normal cells grow most rapidly in the bowel, hair roots, stomach, and bone marrow. This is why you may lose your hair, have diarrhea and nausea. Bone marrow produces white blood cells, which fight infection. Since their number is reduced, you are particularly vulnerable to infections and should report any fever to your doctor immediately. Bone marrow is the assembly line for red blood cells. If your count drops, you could get anemia with symptoms of shortness of breath, weakness, and a general tired feeling. If you tire easily, be prepared for rapid mood swings, including irritability or depression. A drop in blood count also results in your bruising easily, getting a rash of little blood blisters under your skin, or even internal bleeding. A small cut may take a long time to stop bleeding or heal.

If you are still menstruating, you may have irregular periods or stop menstruating altogether for a time. Some women become permanently infertile. Others get pregnant even while taking chemotherapy. Talk to your doctor about birth control, especially since the drugs could have harmful effects on a fetus.

Some drugs affect muscles, making you feel weak or tired. Occasionally there is numbness, tingling, or burning in the hands and feet, but these effects are only temporary.

Hair loss can be the most difficult side effect for many women to accept. One said "Undoubtedly the most devastating side effect of my chemotherapy—even worse than the nausea—was losing my hair. That may sound ridiculous. But I don't think you realize how much hair is a part of your identity until you lose it. When it falls out, it's like watching your body disintegrate before your eyes."

There are remedies for controlling all the side effects, even hair loss. Excellent wigs and hair pieces are available, and as medical expenses they may be covered by your medical insurance. One researcher found that wearing an ice cap over your head while receiving chemotherapy keeps the drug from reaching your scalp and thus decreases hair loss. This is effective, but only for fast-acting drugs. A cap would be impractical, for example, against an agent that is taken over a two-week period.

If you buy a wig, it is wise to do it before you start your treatment. Another good suggestion is to have your hair cut short. Some consolation may come from the fact that the loss is temporary; it will grow back after therapy is discontinued, sometimes looking better than before the chemotherapy.

Nausea may be relieved with medication and by eating small amounts of food more often, eating favorite foods, or bland foods that are easily tolerated, and using liquid protein supplements. Some people have found soda crackers or a dry baked potato without butter helps to relieve nausea. Feel free to try anything you find to be helpful.

Ask your doctor or nurse if you can experiment with the times of the day when you take your treatment and antinausea medicine. Some women say they have the fewest side effects when they take their treatment and antinausea medication early in the morning; others do better taking it late in the day along with antinausea medicine and a sleeping pill.

Some hospitals and medical centers have received approval to give marijuana tablets—actually the chemical THC (tetrahydrocannabinol)—to patients on chemotherapy who are suffering from nausea. But since paperwork is so difficult to process, some doctors say that it is easier for you to get the drug through your own contacts.

Blood samples will be taken frequently to monitor the effects of chemotherapy on your bone marrow and warn of early signs of toxicity.

Another side-effect of chemotherapy is its long-term emotional toll. One study looked at sexual and family relationships, financial situations, and overall activities in women receiving drugs. By the end of the year of treatment, only 12 percent of women receiving drugs could report a return to their previous level of activity. By the end of 18 months, the vast majority had resumed their previous lifestyles. The hope is that drugs will soon be available with less toxic effects and fewer emotional problems.

Back in 1972 I wouldn't have received chemotherapy because it was being given only to seriously ill patients; if I developed my tumor today, I still wouldn't be a candidate for adjuvant chemotherapy because my nodes were free of cancer. Sometimes I can't help wondering what else would be different about my treatment were my disease to occur now rather than ten years ago.

After giving the matter considerable thought, I know my first choice of treatment would be radiation therapy. I know that I would not have made this same choice a year ago, because even then radiation looked too experimental to me. Today, it still would not be an easy decision as I know there could be long-term complications. Ironically, however, like many women treated ten years ago, I received 5,000 rads of radiation after my mastectomy solely for preventive therapy against cancer reappearing on my chest wall. The amount is close to what is used currently to treat the breast after a tumor has been removed. I suspect that if serious or significant complications were present they would have shown up already in women like me who received prophylactic radiation or in the thousands of women who have been routinely treated with radiation in England and France. I could be wrong, but what it comes down to is that every kind of treatment offers some risk. At least radiation therapy offers more benefits than most.

If I weren't a good candidate for radiation, my next choice would be a total mastectomy with axillary dissection and immediate reconstruction. This option would be especially inviting if I were fortunate to live in an area where doctors have obtained good results performing the mastectomy and reconstruction in one operation. I might need to have the reconstruction adjusted in a later procedure, but then I had to have adjustments made even when it was done in steps.

When I received the five weeks of radiation therapy aimed at destroying any cancer cells that might have remained after my mastectomy, I didn't know that a little more than a year earlier a major study on more than 1,000 women from twenty-five institutions had concluded that this treatment really wasn't worthwhile. Women who received the radiation did have fewer recurrences of cancer in their armpit and chest wall, but it didn't affect their survival rates any more than if doctors had treated the recurrences when they appeared. The women studied tended to live as long as those who didn't receive the extra therapy.

Vincent DeVita, director of the National Cancer Institute, agrees with the finding that there is no reason to offer routine radiation to women after surgery. If nodes contain cancer, you should be put on chemotherapy; if they do not, there is no reason for treatment.

Today, there would be near unanimous agreement that I didn't need the radiation. It was easy therapy to go through but increased the chance that my arm would swell and made my later reconstruction virtually impossible without the addition of new healthy skin.

However, to say that nobody needs radiation after surgery would provoke considerable debate among the most knowledgeable people in the field. Controversies exist mainly over women with large, hard-to-remove tumors and those whose tumors are located in the inner section of their breasts. These tumors tend to spread into the lymph nodes along the breastbone—the internal mammary nodes. When cancer specialists suspect that these nodes are involved, they are likely to recommend radiation and possibly chemotherapy. DeVita says more studies are needed to determine whether these special categories of women are benefiting from radiation. But he adds emphatically, these women make up a minority of breast cancer patients and radiation therapy should not be offered routinely after surgery.

Women who have a modified mastectomy or their lymph nodes removed after a lumpectomy will not find arm swelling (edema) as severe a problem today as it was following the radical mastectomy. However, arm exercises are still recommended after surgery to help relieve stiffness and to prevent formation of adhesions (fibrous tissue) which could later limit movement. The exercises, which can be demonstrated by a volunteer from the American Cancer Society's Reach to Recovery program, start with gently squeezing a ball and brushing your hair, then progress to walking your fingers up the wall and twirling a jump rope attached to a doorknob.

I remember after surgery asking the doctor when my arm swelling would go down. "It could take a while," he said. "How long is a while?" I asked. "Some women have had it clear up after as long as seven years," he told me. The fact is if swelling persists for several weeks after surgery it rarely will go away. It means that your operation or possibly radiation disrupted the lymphatic system, which normally drains fluid from your arm.

Although it isn't likely to clear up totally there are several techniques for keeping the swelling under control. Keeping your arm elevated helps, whether you rest it on pillows while sleeping or raise it over the low back of a chair while sitting. An elastic sleeve can also help you get it under control. Some women have success with an inflatable sleeve attached to an automatic pump, which gradually applies pressure to the arm; however, to be effective, the sleeve and pump must be used routinely, some say at least once daily.

Arm swelling may result from an infection or injury years after a woman has had lymph nodes removed. She will always have to pamper her arm slightly, taking extra care against having it burned or cut. Safeguards include not having blood pressure tests or shots given on the affected arm, wearing gloves while gardening, using mitts while removing dishes from a hot oven, avoiding sunburn on that side. It also helps to carry a purse and heavy objects with the other arm and not wear tight jewelry or elasticized sleeves.

Young women who have breast cancer have to explore the advisability of getting pregnant, another area in which opinions have changed drastically in recent years. Berkeley oncologist Norman Cohen, who researched the subject for his patients, explained that formerly the consensus was that such women should never risk pregnancy because the excess hormones released during pregnancy could reactivate lingering cancer cells. He added, "It now looks as though our concern was based more on folklore than actual evidence."

Several studies show that most women who get pregnant after a mastectomy fare quite well, especially if they wait a few years after treatment before having a baby. In another medical turnabout, more physicians now say that when caught early, cancer tends to be almost as curable in pregnant as in nonpregnant women. The crux of the problem, however, is that breast enlargement during pregnancy makes lumps harder to detect and that hormones released during pregnancy seem to result in an especially "high-grade cancer" that grows rapidly.

I recently received a birth announcement from Ellen, a friend who had breast cancer when she was twenty-five. Five years after her mastectomy, she weighed her risks and decided it was time to start a family. "Even women without breast cancer don't have guarantees that they will be able to raise their children," she said.

A totally different decision was reached by television reporter Betty Rollin, who had a modified radical mastectomy in 1975. Rollin explained that she had considered having a child but decided against it, especially after a doctor had told her there could be some risk and if "his wife had a mastectomy, he didn't think it would be a good idea for her to get pregnant." However, Rollin also made it clear that she might not have wanted a child even if she hadn't had a mastectomy. Ellen, on the other hand, had wanted a child so badly that if doctors had emphatically advised her against having a baby, she and her husband would have tried to adopt an infant. There are many possible answers to this problem, but a woman's choice has to be the right one for her.

Once a woman has breast cancer, she has to accept the possibility that a recurrence, stemming from her original tumor, could develop as long as twenty years after her first treatment. However, the longer she lives, the greater are the odds that her tumor won't reappear elsewhere. Eighty percent of metastases—signs of spread—are evident within the first five years of treatment (60 percent occur within the first three years; another 20 percent appear in the next two years).

If you have advanced breast cancer—the disease has spread to your lungs, bone, liver, or brain—treatment strategy changes drastically; treatment is no longer aimed at cure, but at prolonging survival.

Rita, forty-five, and Grace, sixty, who have advanced cancer, are being treated in the same hospital by the same doctor. But each is receiving a completely different kind of therapy. Rita's ovaries were removed as a first effort to stop the recurrence that reappeared one year after her mastectomy. Grace is receiving chemotherapy for cancer spread that was detected only six months after her mastectomy. Who is receiving the better treatment? Actually, each is receiving the most effective treatment for her individual case. Their therapy programs are only two examples of numerous treatments that have to be tailored to the individual.

Rita's breast biopsy showed that her original tumor was estrogen-positive—it thrived on the estrogen produced primarily by her ovaries, but also by her adrenal and pituitary glands. Her doctor favored surgical removal of her ovaries because he wanted to effect an immediate response. He could have decreased her estrogen production by irradiating her ovaries, but it would have taken longer for her estrogen level to decrease. Some doctors are encouraged by reactions to a new anti-estrogen drug called Tamoxifen that enters the cancerous tissue and blocks out hormones. A final verdict on the effectiveness of this drug isn't in yet.

Rita was among the 65 percent of women who benefit from this surgical treatment. Her tumors went into remission, and if the disease follows the usual pattern, will be under control for nine to fifteen months. The period of remission can be even longer. Had Rita developed breast cancer fifteen years earlier, she would have had her ovaries removed *immediately after her mastectomy.* Large-scale studies, conducted in the 1950s and 1960s, showed that survival would be the same if doctors waited to perform the surgery until after cancer reappeared. Now they also know that removing the ovaries will help survival only if a woman's original tumor was estrogen-positive.

As the next step, should Rita's disease recur, her doctor may suggest that she have her adrenal glands removed in order to eliminate another estrogen source. But studies are under way to determine whether a drug* can be as effective as surgery in limiting the hormone production from the glands. As another option she could still receive Tamoxifen. Male hormones—just the opposite of the female hormones her body is used to—would slow down her tumor growth and could be prescribed at a still later date.

Grace didn't have as many treatment options because her tumor was estrogen-negative. Removing Grace's ovaries would not have helped her survive. She was placed on chemotherapy immediately after tests revealed her cancer had spread.

Some cancers respond poorly or not at all to chemotherapy, but breast cancer isn't one of them. Between 60 and 70 percent of the women so treated have a more than 50 percent shrinkage of their tumors. These partial remissions generally last from six months to well over a year. Women who respond to treatment live two to three times longer than those who do not. Ten percent of women will have a complete disappearance of all obvious disease with some patients still free of disease several years after treatment.

Backup strategies exist for treatments that fail or relapse. Success is not guaranteed, but San Francisco oncologist Ernest Rosenbaum said, "It is amazing how often a person who has been successfully treated on a given program and has subsequently relapsed can achieve another remission with a change of therapy. A patient will never know what might have happened unless she is willing to try another therapy, assume the risks, and undergo assessment of the results."

When the treatment becomes worse than the disease, you should have a say about when to call a halt. This doesn't mean you can't change your mind. But there comes a time when the effort should shift from fighting the cancer to keeping you as comfortable as possible. Your community or hospital may offer services that could make a big difference in easing this period for you. Again you or a friend may have to make the phone calls to find out what is available. For example, the American Cancer Society is sometimes able to provide hospital beds, walkers, bedside toilets, and other equipment. If there are enough volunteers, they also can provide free transportation to hospitals.

*(Aminoglutethimide).

To ensure that they can die with dignity some women decide to sign a Living Will (Appendix I). I certainly would want to do so. It states that you do not want to be kept alive by artificial or heroic measures when there is no reasonable chance for recovery. Not only can this statement help you die a more peaceful death, but it removes guilt from your family, who may feel that everything should be done to keep you alive for as long as is humanly possible.

You should also decide whether you prefer to die at home, in a nursing home, or a hospital. Most women would probably like to be at home. If support isn't available, however, and the choice is between a hospital or nursing home, Rosenbaum suggests that the hospital is usually the better choice because most nursing homes need to be upgraded before they can provide the proper warmth and respect for the dying.

More and more terminally ill patients are benefiting from hospice care. Programs are modeled after St. Christopher's Hospice in London, founded by Cicely Saunders, in 1967, as a humane way to help her patients live until they die. Patients can live at the center and go home for weekends or longer. Families can visit at any hour. The atmosphere is open and informal. Patients receive drugs regularly, often before pain becomes severe, and no one worries about addiction. Modern drug combinations are effective at keeping patients free of pain, but alert.

There are many variations of hospice programs in the United States, a great number of which are offered through the Visiting Nurse Association.

The San Francisco area, for example, has at least three such programs. One offers care inside a hospital, another functions in its own building, and a third offers extensive home service from a team that includes a dietician, physical therapist, doctor, pharmacist, public health nurse, and health aides who can visit a few hours a day to give baths or do the laundry, or provide other needed assistance. Again medication is used to keep patients free from pain, but clear headed. For information on hospices, contact the National Hospice Organization; see Appendix G for address and phone number.

Women who would like to understand the reactions of others faced with an incurable disease may benefit from reading Elisabeth Kübler-Ross's *On Death and Dying*. She has documented five common stages that many patients pass through as they approach death, information that can help a dying person understand herself better and provide insight to her family and friends about her feelings.

The first stage is denial and isolation—"No not me, it cannot be true." Kübler-Ross sees this as a healthy reaction, just as it is often normal for a woman who has just learned that she has cancer to respond with denial. She writes, "Denial functions as a buffer after unexpected shocking news, allows the patient to collect himself, and with time, mobilize other less radical defenses."

The second stage is anger; often the visiting family is rebuffed by cheerlessness and lack of enthusiasm. If not understood as part of the emotional stress brought on by terminal disease, these feelings can make the encounter a particularly trying and painful event.

A third stage is bargaining—exchanges made with God for more time or postponement of death. Next may come depression, a time to face reality and mourn over impending losses. The final stage is acceptance, a time almost devoid of feeling, when the patient has found some peace of mind. Kübler-Ross explains that the person often wishes to be alone, requests limitations on the number of visitors, and prefers short visits. Communication becomes more nonverbal than verbal.

Even in the face of death, some women have been an inspiration to others. Marvella Bayh was certainly one such woman. Her life continued even when she knew she was terminally ill. One of the many things she did was write a foreword to the book *Decision for Life*. She said, "The quality of my life actually was enhanced after I had cancer! My values, my priorities were put in order. Love between people became much more meaningful. When you make the momentous decision to live, you suddenly find that you never knew how to live life until you faced the reality of losing it. During this time, I have learned to truly value life, to cherish it, to enjoy it, and to appreciate its bittersweet brevity. So many, many things that seemed important before are suddenly not important at all. You see clearly that even if you lived to be a hundred, life is always too short."

CHAPTER 7

Reconstruction: Restoring the Breast

A forty-one-year-old singer was the first woman to have breast reconstruction. Her German surgeon, Victor Czerny, listened to her concern about not being able to wear low-necked dresses on stage after her mastectomy. He created quite a stir in the medical community when he removed fatty tissue from just above her hip and transplanted it under her chest skin to create a new breast contour. The operation took place in 1895.

With this early start at breast reconstruction, why is it only toward the end of the twentieth century that the procedure is beginning to be offered as an option to breast cancer patients? And even though one million women with mastectomies are living in the United States, why, as late as 1978, had only 15,000 chosen to have reconstruction?

The answer is that, until recently, there were too many barriers—technical, psychological, financial, medical, and even social. Many of these roadblocks have been overcome within a short period of time and, today, virtually any woman who wants breast reconstruction can have it. Not everyone will get beautiful cosmetic results and even the best outcome will never replace a normal breast. But reconstruction does provide a compromise between a mastectomy and a normal breast. At the very least, every woman who has such a procedure will be able to look normal again in her bra or in revealing clothes. For many women, being able to wear a low-cut swimsuit or negligee alone makes the surgery worthwhile.

Some women choose reconstruction because they are unhappy with their external prostheses. A shop owner who specializes in post

133

mastectomy wear told a researcher, "All my clients are unwilling customers. Over 90 percent of them are dissatisfied with the best-fitting prosthesis we can supply."

From my own experience, I'll never forget the "delightful" bathing suit I bought when my mother and I traveled to Hawaii six months after my mastectomy. The blue floral skirted suit with its high-collared neckline certainly was a standout on the beach. At least I didn't have to worry about sunburn. So little skin was exposed.

Some women hate the way the external prosthesis bounces unnaturally against their chests during strenuous exercise like tennis and horseback riding. I have been surprised when a few women have confided that they would rather have both breasts removed so at least they could be symmetrical again.

Reasons for choosing reconstruction often touch deeper emotions. One woman said, "Before my reconstruction I felt more like a victim. That conveys so many painful images, like somebody who has come out of a concentration camp or somebody who was beaten up. Now, I look in the mirror and tell myself that I'm just a woman who had breast cancer. There is a big difference between those two feelings."

Two important studies analyzing why women seek reconstruction came to similar conclusions. One study, conducted by U.C.L.A. nursing professor Sally Thomas, found the overriding concern was that women wanted to regain a sense of body integrity and wholeness. The other study, conducted by psychologist Edward Clifford of Duke University, reported that the primary motivation was for restoration. After conducting in-depth interviews with sixty-five women between the ages of thirty and seventy-one, he found the main concern (55 percent) centered on negative feelings about body contour; for example, feeling unbalanced or lopsided. Thirty-two percent felt self-conscious, particularly when buying clothes or wearing a swimming suit. An equal number believed that their self-concept as individuals and as women had been affected. They did not relate their concepts of femininity to sexuality but rather to how their inner sense of femaleness was affected. They stressed that their primary concerns involved their own sense of femininity rather than what others might think. Seventeen percent experienced strong negative feelings when they viewed themselves in the mirror or while bathing. Only 8 percent expressed concern about their husband's reactions. One woman typified the findings when she said, "I know my husband and family love me. I'm the one who wants to like me better."

Clifford conducted the study because so many physicians suspect that the woman who seeks reconstruction has a "character defect" and is unable to adapt to her breast loss. But he found that the majority of women in his study were stable, well adapted, and quite happy with their sex lives and marriages. He concluded, "Women experiencing mastectomy and reconstruction should not be burdened further by naive speculation about their motivations, their rationalizations, their defense mechanisms, or their ability to cope with reality effectively."

I enjoyed the comment because, of all the barriers to reconstruction, the most infuriating is the reaction that the woman who desires the surgery is somehow weaker or not as well adjusted as one who decides to live with her external breast form.

Since I had my reconstruction, I have seen attitudes change in some doctors; many more, at least in this area, now support the option. In July of 1981, I was told that my county unit of the American Cancer Society was no longer adhering to national policy that didn't allow volunteers with reconstruction to make hospital visits to mastectomy patients. An official with my county unit said she had always questioned the policy, but added, "You know, there were many people who thought something was wrong if a woman wanted reconstruction. Reach to Recovery took a negative view toward the surgery." "How well I know," I replied.

This last year, although the Cancer Society did not permit me to make visits in hospitals, I was part of a state pilot program to evaluate whether women who had breast cancer wanted information about reconstruction and felt they would benefit from talking to those who had had the surgery. The response was yes, something that I could have told them without the survey. As a result of the study, conducted for close to a year in 12 California counties, every Cancer Society unit in California now has at least one trained volunteer who is available to talk to other women about reconstruction. And some units, like mine, are beginning to loosen up on the state policy that still officially says that women with reconstruction might not make the best visitors (a change even from that of a year ago which agreed with the national policy that said women should not make visits). Another sign of change came in November 1981, when the national ACS policy was revised to allow women with reconstruction into the Reach to Recovery programs. I suspect many of the states will develop services similar to the one pioneered in California.

I firmly believe that one reason support for reconstruction has been so slow to evolve is that a breast is involved, which brings up sexual and social images that a woman would not encounter if she lost any other part of her body.

I have heard radical feminists proclaim that women should not have reconstruction because it is only done to please men. Thirty-year-old Judy, a writer for one of the Bay Area's feminist newspapers, who had a mastectomy three years ago, described her mixed feelings: "At first, I objected to reconstruction for myself because it fit into the whole idea of women being sex objects. Somehow I wanted to feel that you could live without it and that you could have a perfectly normal sex life . . . that women are more than their breasts. It seemed politically correct to adjust to my mastectomy.

"Now I see reconstruction as something that would make my life easier. I don't have to keep taking my prosthesis in and out of my bra. The first year after my mastectomy my husband and I went to a campground in Canada, where the shower had no door. I simply didn't shower. I couldn't accept somebody coming in and looking at me in horror. I think reconstruction will make things like that easier for me."

Betty Ford in her book, *The Times of My Life*, said: "Doctors didn't tell me about reconstruction, but even if they had, I don't think I would have wanted it. I felt secure enough with my husband and I didn't want the surgery." The quote is interesting, especially in view of the former first lady's well-publicized facelift. I am not suggesting that there is anything wrong with her marriage or with her choice against surgery, but I think her comment reflects the traditional view that a woman would be more likely to have breast reconstruction if she were not secure with her marriage.

Elizabeth Anstice wrote in *Nursing Times*, "Amputate a leg and the patient is given a costly prosthesis which people hardly notice. Remove a woman's breast and the patient who has suffered a blow to her body image naturally looks for similar care. It seems that many surgeons regard the wish to appear normal as vanity and refer to the prosthesis as a cosmetic aid."

It's difficult to forget the nurse who once counseled me. "Yes, Ann's results are beautiful, but then she's not you. She has had a face-lift already and has had her nose changed. She couldn't live without a breast." This nurse worked for a hospital where doctors contended that most of their patients weren't interested in breast reconstruction. I thought, "The way the option is presented, no wonder so few patients here seem interested."

The fact that the restoration process comes from the area of plastic surgery presents another roadblock for some women. Harriet LaBarre, in *Plastic Surgery: Beauty You Can Buy*, writes, "Many people still view plastic surgery as 'immoral.' Sometimes this attitude has vague religious overtones. 'If God meant you to be otherwise, he'd have made you otherwise.' The normal desire to be socially and sexually attractive [in this case you could add symmetrical] is vaguely equated with sin. People don't want to be thought vain."

In all honesty, I have to admit that I was marginally affected by this view. At first, I felt slightly embarrassed to be seeing a plastic surgeon, someone who does facelifts and makes noses more attractive. My thinking matured considerably as I saw the many accident casualties and young Vietnam veterans sitting in the same office. They could not help what had happened to them any more than I could help what had happened to me. The tragedy is to accept a large scar, when a small one is possible, to live with a deformity when you don't have to.

Equally as important as why some women choose reconstruction are the reasons of those who reject the procedure. Los Angeles nursing professor Sally Thomas interviewed 102 women shortly after their mastectomies and found, somewhat to her surprise, that only nine were interested in reconstruction and of them only five had shown enough interest to have seen a plastic surgeon. Fifty-five of the women said they did not want the surgery and thirty-six said they were undecided. This meant that more than 90 percent of the women were either opposed to the surgery or undecided.

Her next question was, "Why?" The great majority replied that they were fearful that the reconstruction and, in particular, the implants could cause cancer. Because they had just come through one cancer experience, they certainly did not want to do anything to create a repetition.

The next most common reply was that the implant might make it more difficult to detect new cancers. Actually, said Thomas, "There is no evidence that breast reconstruction causes cancer or prevents the detection of new tumors, but these two fears were tremendously important in preventing women from having the operation."

A 1980 brochure from the National Institutes of Health states, "After studying the problem of examining a woman after breast reconstruction, plastic surgeons and radiologists conclude that there is little or no difficulty in detecting an early recurrence beneath or around the implant, using manual examination or mammography . . . Although using implants after surgical removal of the breast is relatively new, implants have been used to enlarge breasts in hundreds of thousands of cases, all over the world, since the 1950s. So far, the Food and Drug Administration and the National Cancer Institute have found no evidence that breast implants have caused any harm."

There are many excellent reasons for women to decide against reconstruction. Nearly 30 percent of mastectomy patients are in their seventies and eighties and may decide against it because of general failing health and financial restraints. Smaller numbers of women in Thomas's study ruled out reconstruction because they "dreaded the possibility of more pain," "feared going under an anesthetic again," "did not want to be away from their families," "felt too old," and "did not want anything unnatural under their skin." But the fact that the overwhelming majority were acting on misinformation makes Thomas question what the decisions would have been if they had had the correct information.

In addition to pinpointing a drastic need for information, Thomas's study found a milewide communication gap between women and their physicians when the topic was breast reconstruction. Nearly 40 percent of the women in her study said they had never discussed reconstruction with their doctors. When asked why, the majority replied that they had not discussed it because their doctors had not brought up the topic. Thomas said, "Many felt that their doctor knew their case, their situation, and the physical results they could expect. They thought that if they had been good candidates for reconstruction, their doctor would have mentioned it. The fact that he didn't meant that he thought they would not be good candidates."

Thomas interviewed numerous surgeons about how they approached the subject. The majority said they waited until the patient brought up the subject of reconstruction as evidence that she was interested. If she did not ask, he would not tell her anything. "There is a tremendous stalemate here, with both persons expecting to get information from the other. The result is that nobody is getting information," said Thomas.

In all fairness, there are some valid reasons some doctors have not been enthusiastic about breast reconstruction. Until recently, results left a lot to be desired for most women. Of all the barriers to reconstruction, the most difficult to break were the problems and poor results associated with the surgery. As recently as the early 1970s, breast reconstruction involved many separate procedures during which large folds of skin were transferred from one part of the body to another. The surgery wasn't covered by medical insurance and could take months or years before completion. Even at the latter stages of reconstruction, serious complications could lead to total failure of the surgery. Final results, reports one pioneering plastic surgeon, could too often be called "grotesque."

A rash of advances made at roughly the same time in the early 1970s changed the outcomes completely. The first breakthrough came with the design of a totally new, soft breast implant—a plastic envelope containing a thick jellylike substance called silicone. Placed under the skin, the implant came close to feeling and looking like an actual breast.

Until this time, breast implants had produced more catastrophies than contours. In the 1930s, plastic surgeons injected paraffin wax under the skin. In the 1940s, fat and tissue were taken from the buttocks, refashioned into a conical shape and inserted in the breast. This left a woman with scars on her buttocks as well as on the breast and, because fat has a tendency to be reabsorbed, the transplants were frequently short-lived. Next came various types of sponges. Some efforts even involved glass balls, and there is one report of a carved ivory implant.

A woman who had one of the early foam implants some thirty years ago recalls, "I faced two months of infection and drainage problems. Scar tissue infiltrated the foam and caused my breasts to harden like rocks. It has been all but impossible to sleep on my stomach." She is happy with the aesthetic results. "But to this day," she says, "I regret that my breasts have lost their sensation. They no longer

The first silicone implants were designed by Thomas D. Cronin of the Baylor College of Medicine in Houston. Unhappy with the high complication rate when sponges were used in women who wanted larger breasts, he first suggested in 1963 that plastic surgeons switch to the new "natural feel" implants.

Reuven K. Snyderman of New York's Memorial Sloan-Kettering Cancer Center went one step further in 1971, reporting that the implants could be placed under skin remaining from a mastectomy. He wrote that the chest skin is far looser and more flexible than had been thought. Equally important, the implant did not interfere with the blood supply to the skin. His paper was received with little fanfare, but many now believe it inaugurated a new era in breast reconstruction.

The first implants came in only three sizes, and a woman had to decide if she wanted her breast to be small, medium, or large. In a short period of time, however, numerous advances and changes have been made in both design and shape. Today, there are three basic types, each available in as many as a dozen sizes and able to fit the A- to D-shaped breast. I will discuss the advantages and disadvantages of each type later, but I must emphasize one point: The implants are not related to the liquid silicone injected into women's breasts in the 1960s. That substance when injected freely into the breast often led to serious problems—droplets wandering throughout the body, getting lost in tissue, sometimes collecting in clumps under the skin and mimicking cancerous tumors. In a few cases, the particles have traveled into the lungs and resulted in death.

The second most important technical event opening the door to breast reconstruction was the move toward less radical surgery in treating breast cancer. When chest muscles were not removed and a good amount of skin was left on the chest wall, an implant could actually look like a breast when it was placed under tissue at the mastectomy site.

Still another milestone came in 1977 at Emory University in Atlanta, Georgia, when plastic surgeons developed a safe and reliable reconstruction procedure for women who had had a radical mastectomy. In an operation that would later prove successful on me, surgeons found they could transfer skin and muscle from a woman's back to replace the skin and chest muscle routinely removed in her radical mastectomy. (The operation, called the latissimus dorsi myocutaneous flap rotation, is described later in the chapter in more detail.) Reconstruction was now available for any breast cancer patient who wanted it and who was healthy enough to tolerate the operation.

Luis Vasconez, now head of plastic surgery at the University of California at San Francisco, was a member of the Emory team that developed the procedure. "The group first became interested in breast reconstruction," he said, "after the young wife of a colleague had breast surgery and wanted reconstruction. The first effort failed, but the incident raised our interest in working on new techniques."

Of all areas in breast cancer treatment, reconstruction is the one that allows women to make the most choices in the decision-making process. The first question to be asked is, Do you want the operation? This is definitely elective surgery and many are quite happy without it. If you decide to follow through with the operation, you have to ask yourself if you want something done to your other breast so you will be symmetrical. Do you want to have nipple reconstruction? Do you want to have a simple or a complicated reconstruction procedure?

Our expectations, priorities, and feelings about our own bodies can make a major difference in our decisions. When I was debating whether I wanted to make a second attempt at reconstruction, I talked with Joan, a woman who had recently had the surgery. At her request, I showed her what I was starting with. "You know," she said, eyeing my remaining right breast, "when you have your reconstruction, you could have your remaining breast enlarged if you wanted to."

"Enlarged," I gulped. "It was just reduced in order to match the implant that didn't take." I liked its new shape. I thought it was a definite improvement. How could I tell her that I never did think large breasts added anything to a woman's appearance? In fact, in my view, the older a woman gets, the dowdier she looks if she has large breasts. She obviously thought differently and was quite proud of her well-endowed results.

The first important choice you have to make is deciding on your plastic surgeon. I can't stress enough the importance of finding the best available doctors, people who have proved their abilities through experience they are willing to share with you. This is not the time to choose somebody who did a beautiful job on your friend's facelift. You want somebody who can do the best breast reconstruction. Experience makes a difference.

Be sure your doctor is certified by the American Board of Plastic Surgery. But don't stop there. Find out what his or her experience with breast reconstruction is.

One way to get the names of specialists is to call the National Cancer Institute's toll-free Cancer Information Service and the national headquarters of the American Society of Plastic and Reconstructive Surgeons, whose numbers are listed in Appendix E and G, respectively. If your family doctor or general surgeon recommends a particular specialist make certain that your doctor has seen the actual reconstruction results of several plastic surgeons.

When you visit the plastic surgeon, feel free to ask questions about every aspect of the procedure as it applies to you. I found out far too late that it was virtually unheard of for a woman to have a satisfying outcome with reconstruction if she had only had an implant inserted in a site that had been treated with a radical mastectomy and radiation. It's easy to say in hindsight, but I doubt that I would have pursued reconstruction the first time if I had known the risk I was taking or the results I could have expected.

Aside from asking the number of breast reconstructions that a plastic surgeon has performed, I think it is an excellent idea to see photographs of previous patients and to talk to women who have had similar surgery. Some surgeons refuse to show women pictures, saying they do not want to create unrealistic expectations and that they may be risking malpractice if the results are not of the same quality.

I was surprised at the number of plastic surgeons who showed me pictures, books, and films when I interviewed them for this book, yet told me they didn't believe in showing before-and-after pictures to patients. If they felt pictures would help me as a writer to understand the process better, why wouldn't the same hold true if I approached them as a patient? Refusing to show pictures is, I think, only setting the stage for unrealistic expectations. Images and Options, the women's group that works with mastectomy patients in the San Francisco Bay Area, advises women who encounter this attitude to find another plastic surgeon.

One doctor told me that he rarely has unhappy patients because, "I take time to tell women about the operation in detail. I outline all complications. I frequently show women photographs of my best results, my mediocre results, and my poorest results so that they have absolutely vivid pictures of the best and worst they could get."

Melvyn Dinner, chairman of the Department of Plastic Surgery at the Cleveland Clinic, believes counseling is critically important in helping women to have realistic expectations and be happy with their final results. In his initial experience with breast reconstruction, he said, 85 percent of women were happy with their results and 15 percent unhappy. Often, there was little correlation between the quality of the outcome of surgery and a woman's satisfaction.

To prepare women better for surgery, the Cleveland Clinic mails information to a woman before her first appointment. It allows forty-five minutes to an hour for the first consultation. Dinner explained, "We also work with women in the RENU Program who have had reconstruction. This gives all our patients the chance to meet somebody who has had reconstruction, somebody who can answer questions about reconstruction that a surgeon who hasn't had the operation is unable to. It's only an impression, but the outcome seems to be that more women are happy with their results."

It is common practice for a plastic surgeon to invite a woman back for a second consultation at no extra charge, giving her a valuable opportunity to ask new questions and to review anything she did not completely understand on her first visit.

Although the selection of a good plastic surgeon is important, several other factors can influence the results of reconstruction. Some you can control; others are difficult to change. The results will be strongly influenced by the type of mastectomy that was done, how much skin was removed, where the scar was placed, and even how the incision was closed. The condition of the skin in the mastectomy area also makes a difference, especially if the scar tissue has thickened excessively or if there has been radiation or a skin graft.

The outcome will also depend on how many operations you are willing to undergo to achieve as "perfect" a result as possible. Once the implant is inserted, even the best plastic surgeon often has to make minor revisions and alterations in the placement and shape of the form. Almost all these improvements can be made under a local anesthetic while you are an outpatient. But because they are inconvenient and produce stress some women choose to settle for less than is possible.

Most doctors want to see how your implant settles before adding a nipple to the reconstructed site or doing anything to your remaining breast. They say the results will be better. Betty, a thoughtful woman who works in an area hospital and who talked to several plastic surgeons even before deciding to pursue reconstruction, said that most doctors she consulted said they would perform her surgery in steps. First they would replace the breast that had been removed by her mastectomy. Next, because she was so large breasted, they said they would reduce her remaining breast to achieve symmetry and, at the same time, reconstruct her nipple. The only problem, from Betty's viewpoint, was that the follow-up operation also would have required a second general anesthetic. "I really didn't want to do that," she said. "I feel awful coming out of an anesthetic and I always think I am going to die when I go under. I chose a plastic surgeon who agreed to do everything all at once. I'm happy with my results, although the nipple isn't centered correctly and I know I would have gotten better results by having my reconstruction done in two stages."

The best time to plan for reconstruction is before, rather than after, the mastectomy. Plastic surgeons have told me that their "ideal" candidate comes in for a consultation before her mastectomy, an option made possible by separating the biopsy and mastectomy procedures.

Fred Tomlinson said that when a patient asks him to consult with her general surgeon before her mastectomy, he advises that a horizontal or an oblique incision, placed as low as possible, be used in closing the wound. When a woman is wearing revealing clothing, these scars are less visible than those that are high and vertical.

Tomlinson added that he also would suggest a general surgeon use a subcuticular stitch—a surgical stitch that runs under the scar, neatly bringing the skin together. Because it saves time, he said, most general surgeons close an incision with a ladder, crisscross stitch, which leaves a scar that is almost impossible to conceal during reconstruction.

Before one sixty-year-old woman had her mastectomy in 1981, her surgeon asked if she were interested in reconstruction. Since her answer was a definite yes, the doctor said he would leave additional skin, which would help her have a more natural-looking breast when she had her reconstruction six months later. The option can be offered to many women, yet it is another example of something that must be discussed before a mastectomy.

Some women have also asked that a general surgeon and a plastic surgeon use a team approach during a mastectomy. The general surgeon performs the mastectomy and the plastic surgeon takes over to close the incision. Realistically, this may never be routine, simply because there are not that many plastic surgeons to assist at mastectomy operations. It also takes careful scheduling, and some doctors may refuse to cooperate because of intraprofessional rivalry. One plastic surgeon told me, "I can see some general surgeon saying, "If I can start the operation and remove the breast tissue and tumor, I can certainly close the incision.'"

If you start with a total or a modified mastectomy, you should get acceptable if not quite stunning results. For a restored breast contour, you need only have an implant inserted under your remaining chest muscles. The operation takes between one and two hours, and the hospital stay is two days.

Lynn, a 50-year-old woman from San Francisco who had her reconstruction a year ago, laughed as she recalled taking off her bandages from her surgery. She removed them in an exclusive lingerie store where she had just spent a good twenty minutes selecting the French knit bra she wanted to wear home. "I was in tears," she said. "There was no way that the reconstructed breast would fit into the bra. It looked so flat and funny. I said to myself 'You went through that surgery for this?'" She called her plastic surgeon to learn that he had neglected to tell her that all implants look flat when the bandages first come off. It takes a few weeks for the substitute to start looking like a rounded breast and a good five to six months for it to assume its final shape.

The radical mastectomy presents the greatest challenge to a plastic surgeon. Although this operation is no longer routinely performed, many thousands of living women have had the surgery. A successful outcome depends on restoring the chest area with new skin and muscle tissue from another area of the body. This extra muscle and skin usually come from the back. The latissimus dorsi muscle and overlying skin are extremely dependable and surprisingly easy to rotate. The body hardly notices that the muscle has been moved.

The new muscle replaces those removed by the radical mastectomy and often can pad the hollow where tissue was removed near the armpit. The new skin provides several inches of cover for the previously tightly drawn chest wall. Even with all the padding, an implant is always placed under the area, usually at the same time that the muscle and skin are rotated. You will have a scar on your back. It can angle down so you can wear a low-backed swimming suit or evening dress or can be placed horizontally so that the scar can be hidden under a bra or a bikini line. It takes about four hours to complete this operation, with a hospital stay of between four and six days.

A few plastic surgeons are enthusiastic about rotating the stomach muscle (the rectus abdominus) and an overlying island of skin for extra padding. It's called the "tummy tuck" reconstruction because you end up with the same line across your stomach as the one resulting from an actual tummy-tuck operation for excess abdominal skin, said G. Patrick Maxwell, plastic surgeon at Eastern Virginia Medical School, one of the first in the country to try the procedure. He believes that it is a good second choice to using the back muscle. "Instead of having a defect on your back, you end up with an asset on your stomach. It's great if the woman needs a tummy tuck anyway," he said. Some plastic surgeons caution, however, that it is more difficult to compensate for and recover from a rotated stomach muscle than from a rotated back muscle.

Ruth is a good example of a problem women can encounter with breast reconstruction. A forty-year-old extremely depressed black woman, she was referred to the Cancer Society and then to me by her social worker. During the past year and a half she had had a mastectomy and two reconstructive flap rotations. Wavering between tears and anger and amid threats of suing her plastic surgeon, she explained: "I had cancer and had a mastectomy and later flap rotation on my right breast. I don't have any complaints about it. Then I was told that I was at high risk of getting cancer in the other breast. I was scared and agreed to a mastectomy and immediate reconstruction. I was told I would only have a little scar under the second reconstructed breast, but they did the larger flap rotation; I still don't understand why. I have no way to prove it, but another doctor was visiting the hospital during my surgery, and I think they used me as a demonstration."

One of the reasons for her depression was that the second seven-inch scar across her back had overgrown badly, or keloided, during her healing process, resembling a thick ropelike line going across her back. For unknown reasons, keloids are more likely to occur in black women than in white.

The lessons to be learned from the handling of Ruth's case are the more involved the operation, the greater the chance of complication. And find out beforehand your chances of waking up with a type of surgery you weren't prepared for.

A few plastic surgeons in the country feel these flap rotations should be done on virtually every patient, including those with the

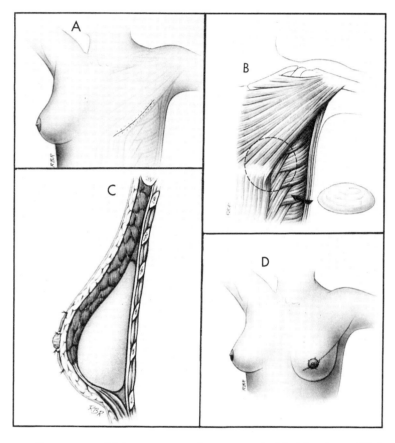

Most women with breast cancer today are treated with either the modified radical mastectomy (A) or the total mastectomy with axillary dissection. Their reconstruction usually involves inserting a saline- or silicone-filled implant (B) beneath their remaining chest muscles (C). They also have the option for nipple areola reconstruction (D). The result lets them look normal in virtually any style of clothing. (Pictures from "Postmastectomy Breast Reconstruction," *Current Problems In Surgery*, vol. 17, no. 11, Chicago: Yearbook Medical Publishers, Inc., November 1980.)

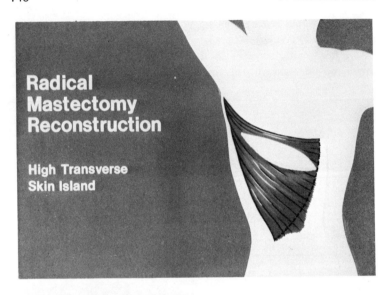

**Radical
Mastectomy
Reconstruction**

**High Transverse
Skin Island**

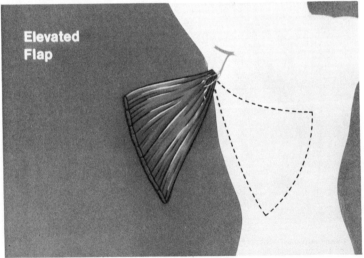

**Elevated
Flap**

The woman who has had a radical mastectomy, and in some cases, the woman who has had a modified radical mastectomy, will need new skin and muscle for a good reconstruction. The tissue is most likely to come from the back area. Here, the latissimus dorsi muscle with an overlying island of skin are

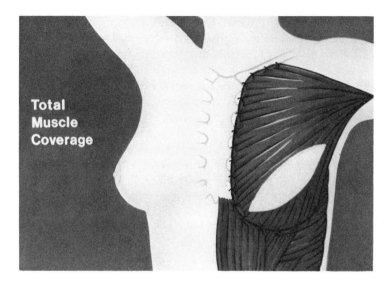

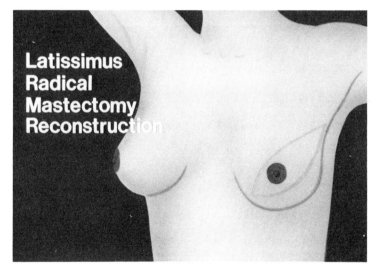

rotated to the chest area; an implant is inserted beneath the muscle and a nipple area is reconstructed. Some plastic surgeons perform all the steps in one operation; other plastic surgeons prefer to reconstruct the nipple area at a later stage. (Pictures courtesy G. Patrick Maxwell, Eastern Virginia Medical School.)

modified radical mastectomy. Most plastic surgeons say they would resort to this procedure on a woman who has had a modified radical mastectomy only if she were missing skin, had had her chest muscle removed, or the nerve to her chest muscle had been damaged. Some women choose this procedure because they don't want any surgery done to their remaining normal breast and are told that the flap rotation will provide a better natural match, especially if their remaining breast is large and drooping.

You're quite likely to find considerable differences of opinion over how much surgery you actually need for a successful breast reconstruction. The best advice I can give is always to get a second or third opinion before proceeding with this elective procedure—especially if flap rotation has been suggested. It's a lot to go through if you don't have to. It's better to have the information before, rather than after, your operation.

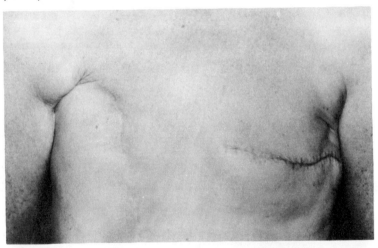

When this woman was 36 years old, her right breast was removed with a radical mastectomy, an operation that removed both of her chest muscles and left a vertical scar. Two years later, a new cancer developed in her left breast and she had a modified radical mastectomy, an operation that didn't remove as much skin and which left her chest muscles intact and resulted in a horizontal scar.

Why would a plastic surgeon do more than is necessary? For a few, money might be the motivation. However, Fred Tomlinson said there is a trend among plastic surgeons today to do the most elaborate, exquisite procedures possible even though they aren't always necessary. "The larger operations are simply more interesting and challenging," he said. "Just as some general surgeons get stuck in a rut thinking that every patient needs the radical mastectomy, so some plastic surgeons see most of their patients as needing the larger flap rotations."

On the topic of implants, there are two questions to discuss with your plastic surgeon: The size and type of implant you want. "I didn't know if I could adjust to the small size of my implants," said one woman who had worn a C-cup bra and after having had both her breasts removed still wore large breast forms. "I looked at the drop-sized

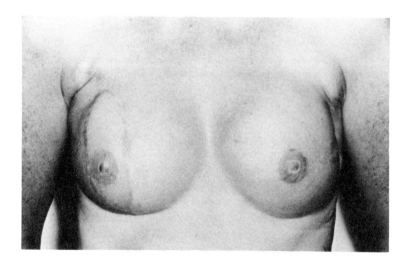

The second picture shows the same woman at the age of 39, following reconstruction of both breasts. As the first step, her back muscle and an overlying island of skin were rotated to her right chest wall. The new skin and muscle were needed to replace tissue removed during her radical mastectomy. In the second step, the implants were inserted. The first two steps required a hospital stay and a general anesthetic. The nipples were reconstructed later (using skin from her thigh) while she was under a local anesthetic. She left the hospital the same day as the procedure took place.

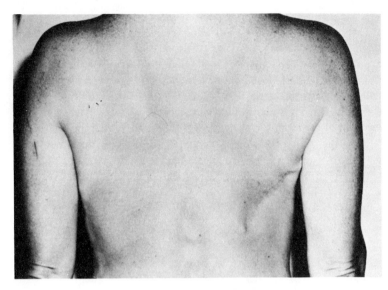

The third picture shows the scar on her back, left in the location where her muscle and skin were taken. (Pictures courtesy Richard V. Dowden, Department of Plastic, Reconstructive and Aesthetic Surgery, Cleveland Clinic.)

implants my surgeon showed me and said, 'Is this worth it?' " To find out if she could adjust, she invested in two $3.50 size-A falsies and wore them for three weeks prior to surgery. She went ahead with her surgery and is extremely enthusiastic about her results.

Another woman I know, however, had just the opposite concern and wasn't so happy with her outcome. She felt devastated when her implants turned out to be larger than expected and went through a second operation to have them reduced. Communication with the plastic surgeon beforehand might have solved this problem. Some plastic surgeons ask you to bring in a favorite bra before the operation and put the selected implant inside the bra to help you have realistic expectations.

There are three main styles of implants available: One is filled with saltwater (saline), the second with silicone gel, and the third, a combination called the "double lumen" implant, contains a chamber of silicone gel within a shell of saltwater solution.

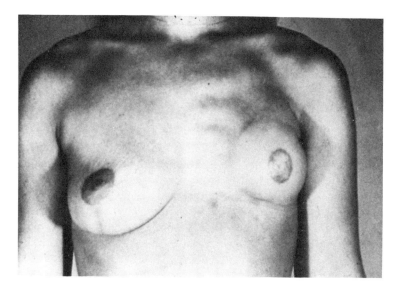

Results can never be guaranteed: This 29-year-old woman had a left modified radical mastectomy and delayed reconstruction. Her implant migrated upward and scar tissue formed around it, causing the implant to contract. Her nipple was "banked" in her groin area for future reconstruction, but lost its color and natural erection after being transplanted to the new breast mound. Complications like these can often be improved on an outpatient basis while a patient is under a local anesthetic. This woman also had her right breast reduced (note anchor- or T-shaped scar from nipple to underfold of breast) to match her reconstructed breast. (Picture courtesy of Washington, D.C., RENU program.)

The silicone implant feels closest to the natural breast. Disadvantages: Minute quantities of the silicone migrate out of the shell. If you place one of these implants on a paper towel for a few weeks, the towel develops a greasy spot from the weeping of the gel. So far, there is no indication that these migrating molecules of silicone cause any harm in your body. Once inserted these implants cannot be inflated or deflated. If a woman has an accident or suffers a severe blow to her chest, the implant could rupture, spreading gel throughout the area.

The saltwater-filled implant can be inflated to the best size at the time of surgery. Minor volume adjustments can be made later by reopening the incision and removing water through the self-sealing safety valve of the implant. If there is leakage through this implant membrane, the body easily absorbs the harmless water solution. The disadvantage of this implant is that because its self-sealing valve does not always close perfectly, there can be immediate or delayed leakage.

The double-lumen implant, the most popular choice today, is a combination of the other two: a silicone core surrounded by saltwater. Plastic surgeons can achieve excellent results with all these products, but they also are the first to admit that the perfect implant has yet to be developed.

There will always be a certain number of problems with medical implants, whether they be a heart valve, a pacemaker, an artificial bone joint, or a breast implant. The main complication with breast reconstruction comes from scar tissue forming around the implant, part of the normal healing process. Problems develop when too much tissue forms and the scar fibers begin to squeeze the implant, making it look rather like a distorted tennis ball. This happens in an estimated 20 percent of cases, more often with gel- than with saline-filled implants. Nobody knows the cause, and to add to the mystery it has been known to occur in one but not in the other breast of a woman who has had both breasts removed. It also can occur months or even years after a reconstruction operation.

If it happens, the doctor can interlock fingers firmly around the implant and manually break the scar fibers. A reported 12 percent complication rate includes everything from rupturing the implant to spraining the doctor's hand. A surgical option is to open the incision and make a circular incision around the implant or remove it completely and reinsert it. Some doctors believe that routine daily massage of the implant decreases the incidence of contracture.

In addition to infection, which can occur after any surgical procedure, possible complications include a hematoma, the collection of blood in the space created for the implant; dying tissue if the blood supply to the skin is inadequate; poor positioning of the implant; or migration of the implant, either upward or downward.

Once the implant is inserted, the most obvious problem is that the "new" breast does not match the remaining one. In fact, it rarely does. A woman has to decide whether she wants to accept the asymmetry or have her remaining breast enlarged, reduced, or raised. In my case, it was necessary to slightly raise and reduce my normal breast, a process that actually improved its general appearance. Some women object strongly to having a breast reduced and choose to have the more complicated flap rotation procedure so that more skin is available to match their untouched remaining breast. I've always idealized the lean, firm athletic body, so I didn't mind opting for the reduction.

If you decide to have reconstruction, you may be asked if you would like to decrease the chances of developing breast cancer in your remaining breast by having a prophylactic mastectomy. As mentioned in Chapter 3, some women also consider this option if risk factors indicate that they have a high chance of developing the disease in their lifetime.

Most women who choose this procedure have a subcutaneous mastectomy, an operation that spares the nipple, but removes between 85 to 95 percent of the inner core of the breast. Some doctors worry about breast cancer developing in the 5 to 15 percent of remaining tissue which, although unusual, has happened in six of 1,200 cases according to one study. For that reason, some doctors suggest a total mastectomy, also called a simple mastectomy. The operation has a lower complication rate and removes breast skin and underlying tissue, including tissue under the nipple area. In both of these operations, the breast contour is often immediately restored with the insertion of an implant under the chest muscle and remaining skin.

Whether to have this operation is your decision, but you should make your choice fully aware that even the experts vary widely in their views about who is a good candidate for the prophylactic mastectomy.

San Francisco plastic surgeon Vincent Pennisi, one of the strongest advocates of the surgery, lists six categories that help him identify a good candidate. He may suggest it for a woman with multiple, persistent breast nodules, one who has had a breast biopsy that produced commonly agreed upon precancerous growths (and some that are suspected of being premalignant); one with a family history of breast cancer (or of other cancers that are linked with breast cancer); a woman who is increasingly anxious about the disease or has already had cancer in one breast and nodularity or cystic disease in the opposite breast; or a person who has had a suspicious mammogram.

Even he cautions that "The operation is at no time to be considered as one to improve the appearance of the breasts. It may well accomplish that end, or it may lead to a disastrous distortion of the breast with severe scarring, nipple loss and skin loss. [Loss of skin and nipple sensation always occurs after the operation, in some to be regained, in others never to return to normal.] The purpose is to prevent breast cancer in a patient who is in a moderate- or severe-high-risk category. The aesthetic results, although important, should never compromise the completeness of the operation."

Because of the potential complications and, more important, because it is difficult to know who will actually develop breast cancer, Pennisi's criteria contrast sharply with those of San Francisco surgeon Thomas K. Hunt. His four categories include a woman with a family history of close relatives who had cancer occur in both breasts; one who has had one breast removed and whose pathology report found multiple (multicentric) cancers located throughout her breast indicating a high probability of spread or occurrrence in her second breast; a woman who has a major lifetime risk, say, who has had numerous chest x-rays for tuberculosis; someone who already had breast cancer and, at the time of reconstruction, decides she would like a prophylactic mastectomy because of a past history of numerous biopsies, because her breast is especially difficult to match or, perhaps, because she wants a complete image change to larger-sized breasts.

There are at least two reasons doctors don't like to recommend the procedure for women who complain of painful lumpy breasts: first, because the pain is usually related to cystic disease, which often disappears after menopause, and second, because in some cases the pain has persisted after the breasts have been removed, suggesting an underlying rib disorder rather than painful breasts.

Rita is a classic example of a woman who has benefited from her choice to have a subcutaneous mastectomy. Forty-five years old and the mother of two sons, both not yet teenagers, she went to a surgeon in 1978 with a suspicious breast lump. The lump was biopsied and, although not cancerous, was "highly abnormal," containing atypical cells which indicated she had a higher than average risk of someday developing breast cancer. She explained, "I was becoming a nervous wreck. Both my mother and my grandmother had breast cancer. After my biopsy, cysts continued to develop. Every time I examined myself there was something new. It was frightening. I used to be a nurse and have seen what cancer can do. I wanted to be able to raise my two children."

She told me that following her surgery, she had not lost the sensation in her skin and nipples and described her new breasts as soft, natural, and uplifted like those of a young woman. But she stresses that she would not consider the operation cosmetic surgery. "The woman who enters this for cosmetic reasons, rather than for preventative treatment of breast cancer, is making a mistake," she warns.

Would she recommend this operation to other women? Rita replied, "I can't give you a yes or no answer. It is up to the woman to decide how important it is to know that her chances of developing breast cancer are markedly reduced. I made the best decision for me."

What would be my personal choice? I am becoming increasingly aware that I do fall into a high-risk group. But I find it difficult to accept the theory that having my second breast removed will make a big difference in my long-term survival. Frankly, I am much more concerned about a recurrence in an organ I have little control over—lungs, brain, bone, or liver—than I am about having a recurrence in my second breast. I wonder if we have gone full circle from excessive surgery for cancer treatment to excessive surgery for cancer prevention. If I accepted the prophylactic mastectomy as a reasonable choice for preventing breast cancer, I ask myself, "Why not continue and have one lung removed, maybe my ovaries, my thyroid?" I must be able to do without several other body parts that are also at higher risk of getting cancer as a result of my personal history of breast cancer.

The decision could be easier for me because I am not plagued with a lumpy breast that requires frequent biopsies and constant worry that the lump might be cancerous. I may come to regret my decision and, as I acquire more information to help me understand what my actual risk is, I may change my mind. For now, however, I fall into the group that prefers close follow-up and vigilant self-examinations over a possibly unnecessary mastectomy.

A woman also has to decide whether she wants to have the nipple complex reconstructed, a process that involves designing both the nipple area that projects and the areola, the darker pigmented area surrounding the nipple. In my view, something is better than nothing, and the creation of a colored circular area is yet another step that makes the reconstructed mound more closely resemble an actual breast. However, in my opinion, this step leaves a lot to be desired and provides the least realistic results of breast reconstruction. It probably is one reason why so many different techniques are currently being tried. Women often opt not to go through with this step.

One of the earliest efforts involved "nipple banking," saving the nipple during the mastectomy and storing it at the top of the hairline in the pubic region. When a woman was ready for reconstruction, the nipple would be repositioned on the new breast mound. A good idea, but two problems developed. First, in many cases the color lightened considerably during the transfer processes. Second, in one case, cancerous cells remained in the nipple area and were transferred to the groin area and back again to the reconstructed breast. Enthusiasm dropped immediately, although some plastic surgeons still like this technique, if the breast tumor is located some distance from the nipple area and if a biopsy of the tissue under the areola shows that the nipple contains no cancerous cells.

The missing areola can be created with skin from other areas—the inner thigh, the opposite areola, inside the mouth, under the armpit, behind the ear, and from the labia (lips around the vagina.) The choice of donor area depends on the color the plastic surgeon needs to best match the other areola, with darker tones coming from the labia and lighter shades from inside the thigh and inner mouth.

With the areola in place, the nipple can be created by using bony cartilage from behind the ear, a silicone implant, or part of the nipple from the other breast. Some women decide against nipple sharing because they don't want to risk losing the erotic sensation in their remaining nipple, an unlikely but possible consequence.

Ruth, the depressed black woman, had the nipple from her untreated breast split for her reconstruction. As a result, her natural nipple seemed to have sunk into the breast and lost all erotic sensation. The transferred part had lost most of its shape as well. "I'm a young, single woman. Why did he have to do that? Why didn't he tell me that there were other options than having my nipple split?" she said, close to tears. Again, I was shocked at the decision made for Ruth and wondered how many other women would carry similar needless grudges through their lives. If I had had her experience with reconstruction, I think I would have been equally depressed.

One reason breast reconstruction is an increasingly available option is that many insurance companies now pay for the operation. Three states—New York, California, and Connecticut—have passed laws requiring insurance companies to pay for breast reconstruction. We're still going through a transition period, however, when one has to check carefully, even in these states, to find if the operation will be totally covered. For example, the law in California states that insurance coverage is mandatory only if a woman had her mastectomy after July 1, 1980. John B. McCraw, of the Eastern Virginia Graduate School of Medicine, conducted a special study of coverage and found "a great discrepancy between the stated policies of the health insurance carriers and their actual policies. Many companies say they cover the surgery, but they won't cover the cost of the operation on the second breast for symmetry, or they might pay for the operation, but not the implant."

McCraw added, "Many companies still don't understand that this isn't cosmetic surgery. These women would not be here if they had not had breast cancer. Some quibble about paying because the breast isn't a functional organ. But then they pay for the reconstruction of a nose, which really isn't needed to breathe, and they pay for replacement of scalp, which doesn't have any real function. Things are improving, but we're still in a thrash with too many cases and I'm not certain why it still persists."

McCraw said that some plastic surgeons waive the uncovered costs themselves, but he is worried that others may step back from doing breast reconstructions because of the problems of getting coverage. I wonder if lack of coverage for operating on the second breast for symmetry is yet another reason some surgeons are so eager to perform the complicated flap rotations that often mean a woman won't have to have anything done to her second breast. Be sure to check on your individual surgeon's policy regarding unmet insurance coverage and communicate with your insurance company before having the operation.

Thirty-one-year-old Cathy of Southern California ran into problems. She had refused to have a mastectomy even though her breast contained a rock-hard tumor the size of a lemon. Blonde, slender, and divorced, she finally consented to a mastectomy, acting as much upon information that she could have immediate reconstruction as the realization that she was risking her life by not having the operation. She came through the surgery well, but because her tumor had been so large, considerable tissue had been removed and her new breast was quite a bit smaller than her remaining breast. But that problem would be taken care of during a follow-up operation scheduled six months later. Her second breast would be reduced and a nipple constructed for her implant.

As she awaited her second operation, actually getting excited about looking symmetrical again, her doctor told her that Medicaid had not approved the second procedure. Already emotionally fragile, Cathy was devastated. Her plastic surgeon sent a second request. Still rejected. Another request to her insurance company went out from her oncologist. Cathy called one night, extremely depressed, saying she was a prisoner in her apartment. She didn't want to go out in public looking so lopsided. "This is awful, I feel so unfeminine. I can't wear any of my clothes." (She wasn't exaggerating; the asymmetry was obvious.)

She continued to wait for Medicaid to reply. I heard from Cathy again and hoped she was calling to tell me that her surgery had been approved. I knew there was a chance she might not be happy with her final reconstruction results, but it would be better than the state of limbo she was in. This time Cathy had the bad news that her cancer had spread and was inoperable. Chemotherapy would start soon.

Cathy's case was tragic: a series of misdiagnoses because her doctors had told her "young women don't get breast cancer"; her initial determination not to lose her breast when she got a correct diagnosis. Had she known about reconstruction, would she have had the mastectomy as soon as she found she had breast cancer? Could immediate coverage by her insurance company have given her a little more time to start rebuilding her life? I knew that life might never be easy for Cathy, but it certainly had to beat dying.

One of the most controversial questions in breast reconstruction today is, When can a woman have the procedure? The decision will probably vary with the doctor's choice, the patient's decision, and her individual needs.

A friend who had a mastectomy in her early thirties and would have been an excellent candidate for reconstruction at any time told me, "I wasn't ready to think about reconstruction for at least three years after my mastectomy. For the first few years, even when it was apparent that death was not imminent, it was hard for me to think in very long blocks of time. For me to go through with reconstruction, I would have had to have a sense of 'I think I'm going to be here a while.'

The thought of having to go back to a hospital was awful. I didn't want to go back for anything, not even to get a breast. I even considered staying out of a hospital when I had a baby." Now, five years after her mastectomy, she is looking forward to reconstruction. She said: "I used to ask myself, 'Why have reconstruction?' Then I said, 'Well, why not?' "

In contrast, one middle-aged woman asked her doctor about reconstruction a few weeks after her mastectomy. "He told me," she said, 'Let's wait two years to make certain you're through the critical period of recurrence.' I told him, 'Doctor, if I'm going to have only two years to live, I want to live them with two breasts.'"

Los Angeles psychiatrist Marcia Goin says you shouldn't forget that when women get breast cancer they have to react to the breast loss as well as to their fear of having cancer. What a woman is most concerned about depends on the individual and the time in her life you meet her, she explained. "You don't want to pressure any woman into having reconstruction, because you can't be sure which aspect she is dealing with."

Goin explained that one of her patients looked at the disease as a growing experience, a chance to reassess her life. "She spent the first two or three years after her mastectomy struggling, coping, and reacting to the cancer and the threat it had placed on her life. She wasn't even aware of having feelings about the loss of her breast. Then one day, she saw a woman on the beach with the same breast size she used to have and decided that she wanted to have reconstruction. Ideally, a woman should know that reconstruction is available, have all the information, and feel free to decide for herself when and if she wants to have it."

Reconstruction can be performed in conjunction with a mastectomy, or at any time following a mastectomy, including as late as thirty or more years after the surgery. Some physicians suggest that a woman delay reconstruction for as long as possible, with five years the minimum waiting period. The decision is based on the traditional belief that a woman was cured of cancer if it did not recur within five years after her mastectomy. Now it is known that a recurrence can occur as long as ten years after the mastectomy or even later. Therefore the five-year wait has lost its rationale.

Many offer another view of why this is poor reasoning. "It does not seem right that a patient be considered cured before we extend the benefit of reconstruction," said Robert M. Goldwyn at a 1975 meeting for plastic surgeons. "All patients are dying minute by minute, as, I might add, are all of us. We do not insist on immortality before we treat other disorders. Patients with head and neck operations need not wait five or six years before having their deformities corrected."

Traditional-minded surgeons, however, may still recommend a two-year wait before reconstruction. They know that the great majority of recurrences occur within the first two years after mastectomy. A two-to-six-month period is an increasingly common option. Doctors may require this waiting period to ensure that the mastectomy scar has had time to heal and that the skin has loosened to ease insertion of the implant.

The most debated issue in timing is whether the reconstruction should be performed at the same time as the mastectomy, a relatively uncommon practice. The procedure adds between fifteen and thirty minutes to the mastectomy operation and requires a coordinated team approach between the general surgeon and the plastic surgeon.

Several plastic surgeons have told me they don't like to perform immediate reconstruction because the results aren't as good as those that can be achieved with delayed reconstruction. They say that complications are more likely to arise from tissue swelling, the large size of the wound, and the fact that the mastectomy wound has not had time to heal. They add that frequently these patients aren't happy, even if the results are very good. They think the implant is more difficult to accept because the woman has not had time to mourn the loss of her breast and to know what it is like to live without a breast. She compares the implant to her former breast, instead of to a flat chest wall.

"It just doesn't work; women are just never as happy with immediate reconstruction," said McCraw. "We find that about 80 percent of women are unhappy with the immediate results, even though they are just as good as the results of women who delay. If they wait, even several days, we've found that 90 percent are happy."

The psychologists with whom I have discussed this opinion find it as difficult to accept and to understand as I do. "It's like telling a person who has had an accident, 'We won't reconstruct your nose now. We'll do it later, because then you'll appreciate it more,'" said Goin.

She suspects that the woman who has immediate reconstruction might not be as happy as one who delays because she is dealing with the threat of cancer at the same time. But she also suspects that the woman would be happier than one who woke up from an operation without any breast. Goin added, "When I ask women who have had delayed reconstructions whether they would have preferred immediate reconstruction, it's a unanimous, 'Oh, yes. Then I wouldn't have had to have a second operation, go back to the hospital, relive my mastectomy experience!' "

One plastic surgeon who claims to get good results and satisfaction from women who have had immediate reconstruction is R. Barrett Noone, chief of plastic surgery at Lankenau Hospital and Bryn Mawr Hospital in Philadelphia. "I didn't want to be an evangelist until we had done a screening program and compared women who had immediate reconstruction with women who had delayed reconstruction. We're now ready to publish our results on a group of sixty women, half of whom had immediate reconstruction and half of whom had delayed surgery and who have been evaluated by a certified psychologist. We really didn't find any different results, either at the time of their surgery or six months later. I have to stress though that we were very selective about who got the immediate reconstruction. These were well-educated women who weren't having emotional problems accepting their diagnosis. We told them that we were not giving them their breast back, but only a prosthesis. They were shown pictures and also met another woman who had had immediate reconstruction and they had a chance to see her results."

He said women were rejected for the option if they showed above-average strain or stress over losing their breasts. He didn't consider a woman ready for the immediate step, for example, if she looked at the picture and said, "That's not a real breast. It just looks like an implant under skin."

There is little question that a woman is a good candidate for reconstruction if she is in good physical condition for surgery and has a positive prognosis. If there is adequate skin and the woman does not have other medical problems, the operation can be fairly routine. But what if there are other problems, and what are they?

Medical factors that place a woman at high risk during breast surgery are the same as those that place her at high risk during any other operation. Lung or heart problems are obvious, serious concerns. Obesity and malnutrition are known to be linked to a higher rate of complications. Diabetes and certain types of medication that interfere with wound healing may present serious, but not insurmountable, problems.

Some women think age disqualifies them from reconstruction. "It's fine for younger women, but not for me," one sixty-year-old woman told me. Actually, a woman in good physical condition has no reason to disregard reconstruction.

Tomlinson told me, "Realistically, if a woman in her sixties or seventies came here but did not have a passion for life and just seemed to be waiting to die, I might find it difficult to encourage her to have the operation. But if the patient were enthusiastic and really wanted to pursue it, I would not object. After all, we do facelifts on women in their sixties and seventies because they want to look their best."

Again, it is a healthy sign for a woman of any age to want to be proud of her body and look natural and attractive in clothes. Interest in breast reconstruction is not a sign that a woman is vain or trying to regain her youth or trying to turn into a sex symbol. It is a sign that she wants to regain a natural, normal body contour and restore what psychologists call body integrity.

What about the woman who is receiving radiation or chemotherapy? When can she have reconstruction? Most physicians advise waiting until treatment is completed. Radiation usually involves a six-week wait, chemotherapy as much as a two-year delay. When a woman is on either therapy, wounds heal at a slower rate. Chemotherapy is known to interfere with the defense mechanisms of the body, thereby heightening the chance of and risk from infection. Plastic surgeon Reuven K. Snyderman says, "If the chemotherapy regime is for one year, I prefer to wait until it is completed. If the treatment period is for several years, I will wait four or five weeks after the last treatment to perform the surgery."

Perhaps the most difficult question is, Should reconstruction be recommended for the woman who is at high risk of recurrence or whose cancer has spread to other areas of her body? This decision, like many others in breast reconstruction, is best made by the patient.

Western culture is increasingly criticized for equating a long life with a rewarding one. The special gift given a cancer patient is the chance to build a fulfilling life around the quality of living. Knowing her life may be shortened, the breast cancer patient diagnosed as terminal can begin to set priorities for her remaining time. Only she knows whether breast reconstruction can help her make the most of her life. It will be a low priority for some women, but others may see it as an aid to accomplishing goals in their remaining months, years, or even decades.

CHAPTER 8

Radiation: Saving the Breast

Radiation therapy is an increasingly popular option for women who want to save their breasts. Although the treatment still draws severe criticism, its numbers of supporters are growing rapidly, the most outspoken saying that radiation will make mastectomy obsolete within the next ten years.

Study after study—from Europe, Canada, and an increasing number of medical centers in the United States—agree that, at five and ten years, survival rates for women who have had what is called "conservative treatment" is the same as for women who have had the more deforming mastectomies. Conservative treatment consists of removal of the tumor by surgical biopsy, followed by several weeks of radiation therapy to kill any cancer cells that may remain in the breast.

Vincent DeVita, director of the National Cancer Institute and a specialist in cancer treatment, said he accepts that "up to seven years after treatment, radiation therapy looks as good as mastectomy. It's very encouraging."

Yes, patterns could change, but since most failures follow within the first two years of treatment, supporters expect the results to hold up.

Brenda Winston and Zoe Snyder are two San Francisco-area women who chose radiation therapy. Winston, a sixth-grade schoolteacher in Oakland, was thirty-one when her doctor discovered a small lump less than half an inch in diameter in her breast three years ago. After the biopsy confirmed it was cancerous, her surgeon advised a modified radical mastectomy and scheduled her for the operation within the week. A friend, however, suggested that she investigate other options and try to get more information on radiation therapy. She talked to a counselor from the Berkeley Women's Health Collective, read a book on radiation therapy, and asked for a second opinion from another surgeon, who also suggested a modified radical mastectomy.

But Winston, having considered her options with her husband, told the surgeon, "I don't want my breast removed when there is a choice." The surgeon picked up his phone and made an appointment for her with a doctor in the radiation oncology department for the same day. The radiation specialist told her she would be a very good candidate for the procedure. She started treatment two weeks later, having had her lymph nodes sampled to determine whether she would need chemotherapy. Because her nodes were cancer-free she didn't; indications were she would be an even better candidate for radiation therapy.

She recalls that the radiation sessions were routine and uneventful. Her breast became red and swollen, but the side effects decreased after about six months. Her breast initially became hard, but eventually softened and now feels like her other breast. There was a little shrinkage, because radiation causes fibers to form and contract within the breast, but Winston doesn't even complain about that, saying, "That breast was larger than my other breast to start with anyway."

Although some women complain of being extremely tired during therapy, Winston said she maintained her two-mile jogging routine. The worst part was waking in the middle of the night and wanting to scratch the area because the skin tended to dry out, almost as if from sunburn.

Winston explained that she wanted the radiation primarily for cosmetic appearance. "I really feel that my husband would have loved me if I had had my breast removed and that we would have maintained a good relationship, but I just didn't like the idea of having a part of my body removed, especially my breast, which is an important part. I think that the surgery would have made me a different person. I'm not shy with my body now, but I think I would have become very self-conscious and withdrawn. My body is something I am proud of and I honestly think that the surgery would have affected my self-image."

Zoe Snyder, a forty-four-year-old clinical social worker in Berkeley, also decided that she wanted radiation therapy after her internist discovered a lump in her breast in October 1979. Her cancer was well over an inch in diameter and involved eight lymph nodes. Doctors told her she had a Stage II—plus cancer, meaning they strongly suspected that it had already spread.

Snyder said, "Once I understood how cancer spreads, I could see that removing my breast at that point would not have made any difference. If it had already spread, removing my breast wouldn't have offered me a chance for cure. And if it hadn't spread, the radiation could control any remaining cancer cells. I just didn't like the idea of losing my breast. It wasn't for sexual reasons. I'm a very tough person, but I don't think I could handle a mastectomy psychologically." She added, "I was fortunate; I had wonderful doctors who took me seriously."

After her lumpectomy, Snyder had a few sessions of chemotherapy and then underwent radiation treatment for six weeks before continuing again on chemotherapy. In May 1981, x-rays found that the cancer had spread to her hipbone; she began radiation therapy for her hip and also started a new program of anticancer drugs. "This is bad enough, " she said. "Just think how bad I would feel if I had had my breast removed and then found that it had recurred."

A few points need to be stressed about this therapy: The studies do not imply that radiation therapy offers better survival rates than surgery, simply that survival rates appear to be the same from both treatments. Next, radiation, like surgery, is successful only in treating the specific region where the cancer first develops, in this case the breast. It has no impact on cancer cells that have escaped to other areas of the body. These are best treated by chemotherapy and various types of hormone manipulation. Prime candidates for conservative treatment who get the best results are usually women who find their cancer early, when it is small—another good reason for practicing routine breast self-examination.

Early breast cancer (Stage I or Stage II) today accounts for 85 percent of women with the disease. Some women with more bulky tumors (Stage III) have been treated with good cosmetic results. However, these large tumors disfigure the breast and removing such a tumor in a small breast can be equivalent to a mastectomy, so that mastectomy and reconstruction may produce better results.

Before interviewing doctors at large medical centers on this "new" option, I visited Berkeley's well-respected Alta Bates Community

Hospital to seek background information. Radiation therapist Theodore R. Purcell showed me slides of a woman who had been treated four months earlier. He explained, "You're really not talking about a 'new' treatment. It may be rather new in the United States, but they have been offering radiation therapy in Canada since I was in high school," said the 53-year-old Purcell. "Other countries—France, Finland, and England—have been using it for years too. Here at Alta Bates we've been using radiation as primary therapy for breast cancer for more than thirteen years. There is always at least one patient going through the program."

The slide that Purcell held to the light showed a picture of two breasts, one a little smaller than the other, but overall healthy and normal looking. Remembering how my chest wall looked after my radical mastectomy, I couldn't believe that this woman and I had been treated for the same disease. It was like stepping into a time machine. How could there have been this much improvement in so short a period of time? I asked myself, "How could a woman of any age not feel better about her body, her life, her future, emerging from a bout with cancer virtually untouched, instead of emerging deformed? Yes, I know many women can accept the mastectomy and build a good life, but why accept it when there are better options?"

With this drastic difference in treatment results, and with many experts saying there are no differences in survival patterns, the obvious question was why it had taken so long for the word to filter out.

"We only get patients when they are referred," said Purcell. "It takes a referral from the physician or interest from the patient to result in change. Basically, it's a job of selling the surgeon. Most breast cancer treatment starts with having a lump biopsied. The chain starts in the surgeon's office. How intellectually honest the surgeon is with the patient determines whether the patient gets an objective appraisal of options. In the politics of medicine, you're talking about referral patterns, money, and egos, and that has nothing to do with what is right or wrong. Remember, this is a surgical country. The theory has been, 'When in doubt, cut it out.' When I finished my residency some twenty years ago, there were only some 230 board-certified radiation therapists. We were a small group without much political clout."

The number of surgeons back then numbered around 20,000. Recent figures show the number has increased to nearly 32,000, while the number of radiation therapists has increased only to 1,500. Radiation therapists are still outnumbered, but today women are demanding to know their options, if necessary by asking for laws like those already passed in Massachusetts and California requiring physicians to outline all forms of treatment for breast cancer to patients. Many doctors still don't support them, but the laws would not have been necessary if physicians had done a better job of informing women.

A vivid description of the problem comes from the statement by Juliet Ristom before the California State Senate Committee on Business and Professions Code. Her experience was the key to California's passing a law requiring doctors to explain options to a woman who has breast cancer. Ristom told the committee, "I was diagnosed as having breast cancer last July. My surgeon—considered one of the very best in Los Angeles—did not think it was important to come to the hospital to give me the tragic information and to describe and consult with me on the surgical procedure he wanted to perform and its possible aftereffects. Instead, he phoned me at 5:15 P.M. while I was all alone in my room, gave me the results of the biopsy, and said that he had the operating room reserved for the next morning to perform a modified radical mastectomy. Even though I was in a state of shock, I had the presence of mind to tell him to cancel the operating room. I also told him that I wanted out of the hospital as I wanted to search for alternative procedures. His reaction was, 'What alternative procedures?'—and I told him that one of them was radioactive implants. He never told me that right in that hospital was the top man for this particular procedure."

She continued: "I will not go into the eleven days of hell I went through interviewing surgeons, radiologists, members of the staff at the University of Southern California Cancer Information Center, and pathologists and reading three of the best books on breast cancer so that I could make an intelligent decision—one that would not destroy the quality of my life, which I felt sure the mutiliation of my body would. I chose radioactive implants and received them from Dr. Ronald W. Thompson at Cedars-Sinai, where the biopsy had been performed. I am not advocating radioactive implants per se. What I am advocating—and am fighting for—is freedom of choice. A woman has the right to decide what she wants done to her body, but if she doesn't know she has choices how can she choose?"

I personally find it sad that the Massachusetts and California patient rights laws had to be passed. Some excellent doctors do outline options for patients. But as long as stories like Ristom's continue to surface, I see no other choice but legislation so that all patients can have a chance to make informed decisions.

Oliver Cope, a long-time professor of surgery at Harvard Medical School, was one of the first to inform women, in his book *The Breast,* that "Mastectomy in any of its forms is on its way out." The replacement: removing the lump—a lumpectomy—and radiation therapy, basically conservative treatment. When I interviewed him in 1979 at a San Francisco convention, he said, "I had to write the book for women because the profession has been so slow to wake up. We doctors aren't educated, we are trained. Surgeons have the longest of the training and it is very hard for them to learn anything new. When you get into medical school you are supposed to weigh what the medical professors tell you and judge for yourself what is the valuable way. But there isn't any time to look at all sides of things, different ways of doing things. You're taught not to depart from what the professor says. 'Do it this way.' Surgery is the worst. You learn that as soon as you deviate, or short-cut or try another way, you may do harm." Cope performed his last radical mastectomy in 1960, after a patient forced him to look critically at the operation to see just what it was accomplishing.

"The woman," he said, "the widow of one of my teachers, refused to have a mastectomy in any form, and made me look at the cruelty of my trade, the surgeon's trade. The cruelty was particularly clear when I realized that radiation following a limited excision could provide an alternative."

Although he didn't mention it in his book, Cope himself put his life on the line with the benefits of radiation only a few years after he performed his last radical. "At the age of sixty," he explained, "I learned that I had a rapidly growing bladder cancer. No one had ever treated bladder cancer with radiation, but I thought I knew enough about radiation that I should look into it. My friends suggested that I have my bladder resected [removed] and accept a piece of plastic as my bladder and have a tube out here and they had a nice receptacle for urine. It only needed to be changed once every ten days. My penis would not have been removed, but it would have had no function. I said I would take the risk of radiation. Now, I am seventeen years past treatment. I don't think I faced a risk."

As Cope wrote in his book, "There are some women who fear losing their breast as much as a man fears losing his penis." Fortunately, women today have much more statistical information behind them than Cope did some twenty years ago.

Wilhelm Roentgen discovered the x-ray in 1895, one year after William Halsted had published his landmark paper on the value of the radical mastectomy. Unaware of the dangers associated with x-rays, physicists soon found their hands scarred and burned. Madame Marie Curie in 1898 announced the discovery of radium, the first radioactive element. Realizing its harmful effects on human cells, she envisaged its future role in treating cancer, but without medical training had no way of applying her new discovery to patients. Her own death in 1934 was from pernicious anemia, the result of years of working unprotected with radiation, according to the biography written by her daughter, Eve Curie.

The first significant attempt to treat breast cancer with radiation came from Geoffrey Keynes, a British surgeon at St. Bartholomew's Hospital in London, who, in 1924, applied x-rays to the chest wall following a radical mastectomy. In 1929, he reported that he could achieve similar survival rates by removing only the tumor and inserting radium needle implants into the breast.

That same year, François Baclesse of the Foundation Curie in Paris began treating breast cancer patients with radiation therapy. In 1939, Vera Peters started her program at the Ontario Institute in Toronto, Canada, almost at the same time that Sakari Mustakallio began his studies in Finland. Most of these early treatments were offered to women who refused to accept mastectomies or to women who were too old or ill to tolerate a large operation.

Baclesse's pioneering work showed that large doses of radiation were most effective in treating large tumors. The problem was that these doses often produced severe complications. But Baclesse also found that complications could be reduced if the doses were fractionalized and delivered over a period of weeks. Sometimes he extended treatment to three or four months. However, his ten-year cure rate for women with early stages of cancer was only 33 percent.

In 1976, Vera Peters reviewed part of her thirty-year experience of treating women with early cancer by radiation and a wedge resection (in which the tumor and a surrounding margin of skin are removed). She wrote, "Concern for the patients' morale as well as their physical well-being has prompted me to present a preliminary report." Peters said the results were comparable to survival patterns of women having mastectomies—a five-year survival rate of 76 percent. Her later reports showed that even at thirty years, survival rates from conservative therapy were as good as those from surgery.

She concluded that if her procedure were routinely available, the more radical treatment could be discussed with the patient and the final decision in favor of either surgery or irradiation could safely be influenced by the patient's special fears. "I would predict that the patient's image of cancer therapists would improve. One might also find that the woman who discovers a lump in her breast would seek medical advice earlier . . . if she were fortified by the knowledge that she did not need to face an extensive and mutilating operation."

Another important five- and ten-year follow-up study of patients treated by lumpectomy and radiation was reported in 1978 by the Foundation Curie. "Our conservative treatment resulted in survival rates at five and ten years comparable to those of radical surgery," wrote R. Calle, director of the Foundation. Of 120 women who had lumpectomy and irradiation, 85 percent were alive and free of disease at five years, and 75 percent were alive and free of disease at ten years.

In Calle's study, women with tumors over an inch (3 cm) in diameter did not fare as well from radiation therapy. To avoid deformity of their breasts their tumors had not been removed. More than half the women needed follow-up secondary surgery, either because the tumor had not disappeared or because it had recurred in other areas of the breast.

Over the years, a series of improvements occurred in radiation therapy to help account for the successful results that Calle and Peters were reporting when tumors were removed. First, studies began to show that the correct radiation dose was critical to good results. Work at M. D. Anderson Hospital and Tumor Institute in Houston showed that women with advanced tumors did not develop other tumors in their chest wall and armpit areas when they were treated with 5,000 rads over a five-week period. Recurrence in the lymph nodes was almost unheard of, even though it was estimated that at least 50 percent of these women had small, nonpalpable cancers infesting the area.

The pattern held up in other cancer patients who received similar doses of irradiation. For example, neck cancer patients with no apparent remaining growths, but with a high likelihood of recurrence, had none after receiving 5,000 rads over a five-week period. Radiation also worked in treating nondetectable gynecological cancers, salivary cancers, and cancers arising in soft tissues—connective, bone, or muscle.

Eleanor D. Montague of M. D. Anderson Hospital, one of the early advocates of conservative treatment in this country, explained: "It became obvious that radiologists had been erroneously concentrating on obvious palpable cancers. For best local control, the focus should have been on removing the tumor with surgery and then treating any remaining cancer with radiation. With modern doses we now know that radiation is 95 percent effective at treating microscopic residual cancers still remaining in the breast."

At the same time that radiologists were improving knowledge about dose requirements, a rapid advance in technology was taking place. Early instruments that left most of the radiation outside the skin were replaced with higher-voltage x-rays and cobalt-60 beam therapy that spared the skin so only mild tanning resulted. The newest form of irradiation makes use of high-energy electron beams, which can be controlled to deposit their radiation in specific depths, thus sparing underlying tissue like heart, lungs, and ribs.

Still, critics contended that there had been no quality controlled random study in which some women received surgery and others lumpectomy and irradiation. Reported statistics were always calculated in hindsight which can bias the interpretation. The one study that could have answered the question was performed at Guy's Hospital in London, from 1961 to 1971. Some 370 women fifty years and older were treated by either radical mastectomy or removal of the tumor and a section of surrounding breast. Both groups received radiation therapy. Five- and ten-year results found no difference between the two groups for Stage I cancer, but Stage II patients fared better with radical mastectomy.

Those who favor surgery frequently use these data to support their viewpoint. However, the study contained several "serious flaws," according to Allen S. Lichter, head of radiation therapy at the National Cancer Institute. He said that women treated by irradiation received 1,500 to 2,000 rads less than are recommended today. Treatments were delivered over a three-week period, instead of over today's standard five-week period. And although the breast lumps were removed, physicians left palpable and suspicious lymph nodes in place. Most recurrences occurred in these nodes.

Skeptics still waiting for a properly conducted and analyzed study are following three today—two in the United States and one at the National Cancer Institute in Milan, Italy. Results from Italy, reported in the July 2, 1981, issue of the *New England Journal of Medicine*, add considerable weight to treating the breast with conservative therapy. Between 1973 and 1980, women whose tumors were under an inch in diameter (2 cm) and whose lymph nodes appeared to be free of cancer were randomly assigned to one of two groups. Three hundred and forty-nine women had the Halsted radical mastectomy and 352 had a quarter of their breast removed as well as some lymph nodes and were treated with radiation therapy.

Umberto Veronesi, director of the study, reported no difference between the two groups in disease-free or overall survival. There were three local recurrences in the Halsted group and one in the group that received the conservative treatment. He concluded, "From these results, mastectomy appears to involve unnecessary mutilation in patients with breast cancer of less than two centimeters and no palpable lymph nodes."

In an earlier interview, he said, "I think too many mutilations have been done because we wanted to reassure ourselves, because we wanted to be in a position of certainty, so we could defend our professional pride. But I think we should consider the point of view of the woman."

Within the next few years, it will be possible to compare his findings to a random study started by the National Surgical Adjuvant Breast Project in 1976 and another begun by the National Cancer Institute in 1979. So far, these studies haven't been in progress long enough to produce meaningful results. However, numerous medical centers, and even community hospitals, are reporting with increasing frequency that women with early cancers treated by radiation are doing as well as those who received mastectomies.

For example, at Harvard's Joint Center for Radiation Therapy, a medical team headed by Samuel Hellman has treated more than 550 women, some 200 in 1980 alone. In April 1981 Hellman said, "At seven years our patients continue to do as well as those treated by surgery. Patients have been followed a minimum of thirty months, an

average of four years, and as many as eleven years after treatment.''
A cooperative study at Harvard, Yale, Hahnemann, and Jefferson medical schools found that the five-year survival rate for early breast cancer was 83 percent and the ten-year rate was 64 percent. ''These results are entirely comparable to the great majority of surgical studies in the literature and reinforce our conclusions that radiation-treated patients and those having mastectomy survive equally well—but that radiation therapy offers the great advantage of preserving the breast,'' commented Leonard R. Prosnitz of Yale.

Although this will never appear in any medical text, I have learned that one way to judge the effectiveness of a treatment is to become aware of who is recommending it. For example, most plastic surgeons were extremely enthusiastic about breast reconstruction—after all, that is their specialty. But I felt it a sure sign their results were improving when I heard surgeons and radiologists discuss the plastic surgeons' beautiful results. The same is true of radiation therapy. Radiologists have been endorsing it for years, but now, I'm beginning to hear about the benefits of the treatment from surgeons, oncologists, and epidemiologists.

For example, Stephen K. Carter, director of the Northern California Cancer Program, who chaired the 1980 consensus panel on chemotherapy, said, ''If I had a family member with a tumor, I wouldn't hesitate to have it treated by radiation therapy. I am persuaded by the data. It looks as good as radical mastectomy to me. I wish we had fifteen years of follow-up, but if it were a member of my family, particularly a younger person with a small tumor, I would not hesitate to recommend radiation therapy.''

A young surgeon from Chicago said to me at the nineteenth annual Conference on Breast Cancer in San Diego, ''You're writing a book on breast cancer. Well, what are you going to say is the best treatment?''

''I have to say that today, the best treatment is what the woman decides is best for her. There are no right answers. If she wants to preserve her breast and take a small risk because final results aren't in, then radiation seems the way to go. If she wants treatment backed by years of data, then surgery is best.''

He said, ''It's a difficult time. A woman visited me a month ago with a small lump and I performed a modified radical mastectomy.

She came back for a follow-up visit a week ago with an article from a woman's magazine on radiation therapy and asked 'Why couldn't I have had that?' To be honest, I didn't know what to tell her. I didn't know why she couldn't have had radiation."

Although some doctors are quick to criticize women for being vain enough to risk their lives with radiation therapy, the fact is that other forms of cancer are being treated that way. It has been shown that surgery and radiation therapy give comparable results in treating early cancer of the vocal cords. Since treatment with radiation preserves the voice function, it is now standard treatment. Recent results show that primary radiation therapy in early prostate cancer appears to bring the same results as those obtained by radical surgery. Since radiation preserves sexual function, it is increasingly being recommended, especially in young men, as an alternative to surgery, which always results in sexual impotence.

Are patients happy with the final cosmetic results of radiation therapy? Thirty-one patients treated at Harvard over a seven-year period were asked to evaluate their results. Twelve of the women said their results were "excellent," fourteen replied "good," four judged them to be "fair," and one woman said hers were "poor." I had to ask myself, "How many women with radical mastectomies or even modified mastectomies could judge their results as excellent, good, or fair in comparison to their remaining breast?"

Long-term survival and cosmetic outcomes are two factors used to evaluate any breast cancer therapy. A third exists that is equally as important—the rate of local recurrence in the treated breast and in the lymph nodes. Rates of local recurrence in the early studies ranged between 25 and 56 percent, a totally unacceptable number for two reasons: First, it meant treatment wasn't reaching all cancer cells. Second, local recurrence following surgery usually is an ominous sign that the cancer has spread to other areas of the body.

Modern radiation therapists say it is unfair to look at the early studies that produced high recurrence rates because they are based on patients who didn't receive adequate radiation doses. One study was of patients whose tumors weren't even removed. More important, the therapists claim that local recurrences following conservative treatment are frequently not a grave sign. For example, in the Toronto study, 152 women developed local recurrences after having received radiation therapy. Fifty-four percent survived at least five years after recurrence, and 32 percent lived for ten years or more.

When cancer reappears on the chest wall after radical surgery, it generally is suspected of being the first sign of serious systemic problems. After conservative treatment, reappearance in the breast is more likely to be indicative of local-treatment failure that signifies the need for further local therapy. With modern radiation therapy, ominous local recurrence rates range between 5 and 10 percent—about the same as after mastectomy.

Pioneer radiotherapist Eleanor Montague said that twenty years ago it was difficult to find a good treatment center for conservative therapy—only about three existed in all of North America. Now, she estimates the number at between fifty and seventy.

What's the best way to find a good conservative treatment if you want to pursue this option? Several routes exist. You should be able to get the information from the National Cancer Institute's toll-free Cancer Information Service or by phoning the department of radiation oncology at your nearest medical school.

Jay R. Harris of Harvard admits that his center may soon get more requests than it can handle, but added that the number of well-trained doctors in the community is increasing all the time. "Every week we have radiotherapists visit us and spend time in our department to see what we are doing. And we go out and give talks." So even if his center has to turn away women, he believes good treatment exists elsewhere.

Montague said she has strong reservations about the treatment spreading to the community level. "I don't think your friendly community radiologist should do it. Smaller places just don't have the experience of treating hundreds of breast cancers with the breasts still in place. They also aren't as likely to have strong and necessary support services from surgery and pathology. We put our patients through a tremendous selection process. We don't do anything without looking at the woman's mammogram with a diagnostic radiologist. If the patient has multiple cancers, we don't think she would make a good candidate. We work with our pathologist, and if he sees something on the woman's pathology report which makes him think she would not be a good candidate, we tell the patient. And treatment isn't successful unless a surgeon and a radiotherapist work together. It is as important for the surgeon to remove all obvious disease as it is for the radiation therapist to deliver a well-defined dose of radiation therapy."

Montague said that if she doesn't know the thoroughness of work done by a woman's surgeon, she doesn't hesitate to ask that more tissue be removed from the referred patient's biopsy site. As often as 70 percent of the time, she finds these women have small margins of tumor left from the first biopsy, which are more difficult than microscopic growths to control with radiation.

Remember, just as in the case of breast reconstruction, experience counts. Even if you can't get to a center that has a lot of experience, which I think is your best option, it would certainly be a wise idea to ask how many women have been treated at a facility and to find out how much experience the radiation therapist has had in treating breast cancer patients with conservative therapy.

What is the procedure for conservative treatment? Treatment sessions are fairly standard today. Most sessions are given five days a week, Monday through Friday, over a five-week period. Before the first treatment, a radiation therapist will mark your treatment area with colored ink. It's important not to wash off these marks until you have finished all your treatments. They make a target to ensure that the radiation gets to the same place each time. Some of the ink may rub off, so you might not want to wear light-colored clothes or your best things until you have finished your treatments. As you will have to undress for treatments, wear clothing that is easy to put on and take off.

Each treatment session takes fifteen to twenty minutes, with the majority of time spent on correct positioning under the radiation machines. Treatments last only a minute or two. The radiation will be aimed at your breast, but the machine may be rotated to treat your lymph node areas too. The radiation therapist leaves the room when the machine is on, but he or she monitors you through a window or on a television screen and you can talk to your technician over an intercom system. Small amounts of radiation may miss their target and scatter elsewhere in the room. Technicians aren't threatened by levels released during your individual session, but leave the room out of concern about exposure to radiation from many patients for periods of months or years.

It's only normal for a woman to find being alone by herself in a

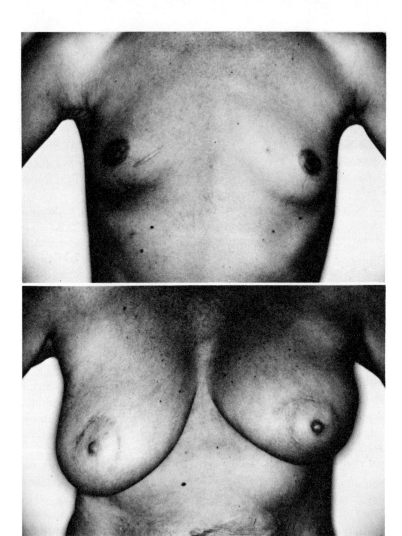

Each of these women chose to have her breast cancer treated by a lumpectomy and a follow-up course of radiation therapy.

The first picture shows a 34-year-old woman fifteen months after she had a tumor removed from the inner area of her right breast and had completed radiation therapy.

The second picture shows a 63-year-old woman one year after her left breast was treated for breast cancer. The tumor was removed from the upper-inner area of her breast. Her treated breast is smaller because radiation caused fibers to form and retract or shrink tissue, a condition that is not unusual in pendulous breasts, especially in older women.

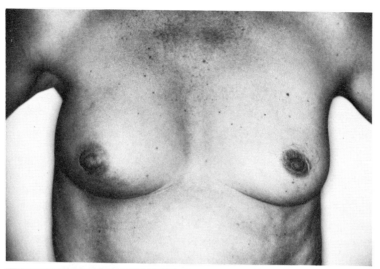

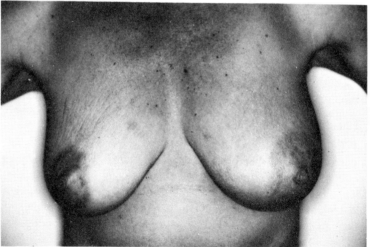

The third patient is a 56-year-old woman who had a tumor removed from the outer side of her right breast. Numerous lymph nodes contained cancerous cells, so she underwent both radiation therapy and chemotherapy. She is shown here approximately 18 months after finishing radiation therapy and nine months after completing chemotherapy.

The fourth picture shows a 48-year-old woman two years after a tumor was removed from the outer area of her right breast and she had finished a course of radiation therapy. She had one positive lymph node involved with cancer, but elected not to have chemotherapy. (Pictures courtesy of Allen S. Lichter, Head, Radiation Oncology Branch, National Cancer Institute.)

room under a large machine a little lonely and frightening. One woman who had radiation therapy told me, "I eventually got used to it, but I was never really able to relax completely." It helps to have something else to think about when you're receiving the treatment. Another recent patient said meditation and mental relaxation exercises helped her through sessions.

As a final step, most centers like to deliver an extra 1,500 to 2,000 rads of radiation to the specific area where your tumor was removed, either by concentrating radiation to that region for another week or two of treatments or by placing thin tubes containing the radioisotope iridium 192 directly through the breast. The tubes can be inserted while you are under a general or a local anesthetic and remain in place for between fifty to sixty hours, during which time you will be confined to a hospital room. The radioactive material is aimed at destroying any cancer cells that might still be in your breast. Radiation is concentrated at your tumor site, but also penetrates through all of the breast tissue. As a precaution you will be asked to discourage visitors or restrict them to persons over eighteen who are not, and are not likely to, become pregnant.

Usually the implant can be removed right in your room, with only a light pain medication required to make you comfortable. When the implants are removed, your therapy is completed and you need only return for follow-up checkups.

Treatments can be tiring. Mild fatigue is the most common side effect of radiation therapy. Don't feel you must keep up with your normal activities. You may have some loss of color in the nipple area. After about three or four weeks of treatment, you may notice your skin becoming dry, tender, moist, or itchy. There are sprays and medications to counteract the skin changes, so ask your doctor about them. Also, don't use creams, lotions, soaps, cosmetics, deodorants that haven't been recommended because they may contain materials that could irritate your skin. For example, talcum powder contains an abrasive. Adhesive tape should not be used because the skin is sensitive and may come off with the tape. Because heat or cold may further irritate your already sensitive skin, don't apply hot-water bottles, ice packs, hot water compresses, electric heating pads, hot packs, or heating lights on your treatment area.

Allen S. Lichter, who heads the National Cancer Institute's therapeutic radiology section, warns that one shouldn't assume that surgery is "hard" treatment and radiation "easy" treatment. "They're both demanding forms of treatment for the patient," he stresses.

Sixty-year-old Ann, a San Francisco woman who had a lumpectomy and radiation therapy a year ago, knows that radiation is not "easy." "My whole breast got so sensitive that I couldn't wear a bra. My skin felt like raw nerves. The worst part was that nobody wanted to admit that the radiation had caused it. I thought I was becoming psychotic." Ann said she tried everything she could think of to control the pain. "I got medication from my three doctors and walked around like a zombie for a month until one doctor decided I should get off all the medication and just take aspirin. I even tried a faith healer and a holisitic health center."

Several months after radiation, Ann said her skin wasn't so sensitive and she expected to be back to normal in a few more months. She started to cope with her problem much better after her doctor explained that her skin had been extremely sensitive to radiation. "I really think I could have dealt with the pain earlier if they had just explained what was happening. I can accept anything as long as I know what is happening," she said. Ann's other problems were minor. She had some difficulty swallowing, probably because scatter from the radiation had irritated her throat. She also had a radiation burn, an open sore, but that cleared up after a week and a half.

In a paper presented at a 1980 National Conference on Breast Cancer, Samuel Hellman of Harvard reported that 20 of 176 women treated at his center suffered early complications; seventeen were defined as having "temporary" or "mild" complications; three had "long-term" and "significant" complications.

The mild complications category included ten patients with rib fractures, a problem that reportedly has been resolved with lowered dose levels of radiation. Five women suffered radiation-induced pneumonia, a real problem but one often so mild that patients don't have to be hospitalized. One woman reported a prickling or tingling sensation of her skin; another woman had excess fluid develop in her chest area.

Significant problems consisted of long-term swelling of one woman's arm and a general arm weakness that resulted from nerve tissue contracting within the shoulder area of another woman. A third patient, who had been treated simultaneously for cancers in both breasts, developed a constriction of the envelope of tissue surrounding her heart. The patient had surgery to have the small fibrous area removed and is now well.

One long-time professor of radiology told me that places like Harvard's Joint Center for Radiation Therapy probably have low complication rates because they have the best equipment and some of the best talent. "When the news breaks that one institution has excellent results with a treatment—be it radiation or anything else—don't think you're going to get the same results in other places that aren't able to attract people at the top of their field," he said.

Remember, most women won't have complications and even Ann says she would still choose radiation over surgery. But you are not talking about a particularly easy treatment.

One difference between surgery and radiation is that the results of surgery—good or bad—are soon obvious. Some doctors are quick to admit their concern that radiation therapy may produce long-term problems for patients, expecially for younger women, "who have the most to lose," according to San Francisco surgeon William H. Goodson. "We have evidence on five to ten years after radiation therapy, but nobody has looked at long-term results fifteen to twenty years down the road. If we give a young woman with a good prognosis and a favorable lesion 5,000 rads, she may have radiation scatter to other areas of the body—the stomach, the esophagus, and thyroid. We're going to feel pretty bad if fifteen to twenty years from now she shows up with a new cancer in one of those areas."

Eleanor Montague reports that in her many years of using radiation to treat women with early stages of breast cancer, only 2 percent developed new cancers in other organs compared to the 1.3 percent of patients treated by surgery who developed additional cancers. The difference is not significant. Second cancers, when they develop, tend to show up in the uterus, colon, or thyroid gland; in more recent years they have shown up in the lungs. However, one radiation therapist said, "We simply have not had enough patients from whom to draw firm conclusions about long-term effects of radiation. You need thousands and thousands of patients and they don't exist yet." Institutions are just beginning to pool information with hopes of answering this question. However, results won't be in for years yet.

Harvard radiotherapist Jay Harris co-authored a chapter on radiation for a 1981 medical book, *Annual Review of Medicine,* that touches on his group's feelings about radiation risk. It states the conservative therapy for breast cancer "was first begun as early as the 1930s [in France, Canada, and Finland], and there have not been any reported second malignancies following this treatment." Although the chapter states that the issue has not been fully clarified, it contends that "present evidence suggests this risk is small."

The chapter notes too that low-dose radiation appears much more likely to cause cancer than the high-dose used in breast cancer treatment. The population of women who received low doses of radiation (500 to 1,000 rads) to control benign uterine bleeding developed a threefold increase in leukemia. Yet higher doses applied to the same area have failed to cause any increased risk. The explanation is that low-dose radiation can in fact cause normal, healthy cells to transform and become cancerous. High doses, however, seem to "inactivate" or "sterilize" the cell, with the overall risk of cancer actually decreasing.

Conservative treatment of breast cancer is likely to produce heated debate for several years. And another issue on the horizon will generate just as much emotion: Is radiation really necessary after a lumpectomy? The important National Surgical Adjuvant Breast Project sudy, started in 1976, includes one group of women being treated only by having their tumor and a surrounding margin of tissue removed. It will provide an answer, but results aren't expected for several years.

One reason progress is slow with new options such as reconstruction and radiation therapy is that both call for re-educating physicians and patients. Change takes time and many women still view these options as frivolous. I suspect these same women, however, would do everything possible to keep a child or husband from losing a body part if there was a choice.

I know a large part of the problem is that women have a difficult time taking themselves seriously. Too many women are conditioned to think of everyone else first, always to give and never expect to receive the best for themselves; in fact, they tend to feel guilty at times about inconveniencing others when their own well-being is involved.

On a recent radio program a cancer specialist was being interviewed when a woman called in to ask about reconstruction. "I've already put my husband through so much, how can I possibly ask him to stick with me through more surgery?" The interviewee replied, "I don't know what you're going to decide about reconstruction, but you should realize that you didn't put your husband through a lot. A disease put both you and your husband through a lot."

There is nothing trivial about a choice that helps maintain or preserve your normal body—especially when studies show that the choices are as good as the more mutilating procedures.

CHAPTER 9

Future Directions

Talking to a group of nurses recently, I was asked by one woman if I were planning on having children. I told her that my husband and I had decided that we would like to have a family. What I didn't tell her, however, was that tests had shown I would probably have to take a fertility drug to conceive a child. I felt the risk from the pregnancy was small and worth taking. But I am still debating about another risk, although probably a quite small one, of upsetting my seemingly safe natural hormone pattern with fertility drugs.

After the meeting, the woman who had posed the question came up and asked, "If you were pregnant and knew you had conceived a girl, would you ask for an abortion?" We both knew that my daughter would have an increased risk of getting breast cancer during her lifetime. I was shocked at the question if only because I know how delighted I would be to learn I was about to have a daughter. But it also gave me insight into how much some women fear this strange disease. Even if I were 100 percent certain that my daughter would have breast cancer, I would never consider an abortion. I shuddered at the thought of my mother terminating my life before it started because she could foresee that I would get breast cancer.

On the whole, I've enjoyed my thirty-four years. I would not want to trade my life and experiences for those of another woman solely because she hadn't developed breast cancer. If anything, having had breast cancer has made me appreciate life more. For the first few years after my mastectomy, my top priority was to enjoy the present. I took every opportunity to travel, not because we had extra money but because that is where we put the money we had. My husband and I flew to Hawaii, Europe, the Yucatan in Mexico, back to Hawaii, and then Ireland and England. We plan a trip to Australia and New Zealand in 1982. We've also seen much of the United States.

I was fortunate to find a job that was challenging but gave me weekends and evenings to do what I wanted—to enjoy my relationship with my husband, to take classes in everything from aikido and tennis to interior design and anatomy and physiology. I also had time to attend plays and dance programs, garden, hike, play tennis, and jog and to develop good friendships. I am glad that I have tried to help others cope with breast cancer, first as a volunteer for the Reach to Recovery Program and now as a resource person on breast reconstruction. There is no question in my mind that, given a choice, I would have preferred never having had breast cancer and never having had to realize just how fragile life can be. I suspect that I am leading a different life from the one I would have if I hadn't had breast cancer, but I really can't say this is a worse one. I would hope that my daughter would feel the same.

Another reason I couldn't deny her life is that I am optimistic enough to believe that by the time she were old enough to have breast cancer, science will have found a cure, will have unlocked the mystery of all cancer. Even if a cure isn't found in the next few decades, treatments will certainly continue to improve. Many of today's frustrating questions will have answers based on results of clincal studies. Experts believe a more detailed understanding of cancer biology will help predict how individual women's cancer cells will respond to various combinations of chemotherapy, surgery, and radiation. Drugs, they say, will be less toxic and have fewer side effects. Most women will probably not be disfigured by surgery. If reconstruction is still necessary, some predict it will be done routinely at the time of surgery, with even better results than are now available.

What are some of the specific new directions?

In detection, efforts are being made to help high school and college age women practice routine breast self-examination. Close to 17,000 students in California have received instruction in a program sponsored by the American Cancer Society. A film on breast self-examination is shown the day before a volunteer team visits gym classes. A Reach to Recovery volunteer shares her experiences, a nurse explains proper techniques for examination, and a surgeon discusses medical aspects.

The Wisconsin Clinical Cancer Center in Madison has developed a class outline for teaching breast self-examination to high school seniors. The aim is to have students make breast self-examination as regular a health habit as brushing teeth. Studies show that women who know how to examine themselves are more likely to seek early medical treatment than those who do not. If new treatment options are presented, women will know that breast loss isn't the price they must pay for finding a lump.

A major breakthrough in detection may come with the development of a simple blood test that could detect cancer years before it could be felt. Right now, a detectable lump consists of as many as a billion cells. Treatment could be much more effective if cancer could be found at even the 10-million-cell level. None of the tests now available are that accurate, but many believe these tumor detectors will some day exist.

The trend is toward diagnostic procedures that are less painful, less dangerous, and involve fewer x-rays. Transillumination is one technique that quite literally shines a new light on breast cancer diagnosis. Light is shown through the breast and the interior image is recorded on highly sensitive infrared film or reproduced on a television monitoring screen. Tissues transmit light differently, and doctors who use the process in Sweden say it can spot small growths likely to be cancerous, especially in younger women whose breasts are more difficult to diagnose with mammography. Researchers in the United States are beginning to evaluate the procedure, which is also called diaphanography.

New treatment areas show promise. A doctor's dream is to be able to predict how well a particular anticancer drug will work in an individual patient. Several groups are investigating tests that may give the answers. Cells from the patient's tumor are grown and subjected to different drug treatments. One such technique, the Salmon stem cell test developed at the University of Arizona, gives an excellent prediction of which drugs won't work in patients and is about 60 percent successful in forecasting which will be effective. In another version of this test, the patient's tumor cells are injected into a mouse subsequently treated with various drugs to determine which will be effective. Tests like these may someday be routine in most hospitals, essentially helping to take the guesswork out of treatment.

Work is under way to help boost the body's own natural defenses against cancer cells. So far immunotherapy has not made a significant contribution, but this could change in the future. The most exciting future direction involves the manufacture of synthetic antibodies. The body's own natural antibodies are a first-line defense against infection and disease. Scientists are trying to mimic the process by creating antibodies in the laboratory that only attack cancer cells. Some researchers are trying to develop specific substances for breast cancer tumors. Work is still very experimental. However in the future, radioactive substances may be combined with these antibodies. The new product could then be injected into the body to search for very small and early cancers. Another idea is to add to antibodies specific anticancer drugs that will cluster around and destroy cancer cells but ignore healthy ones.

Another innovative and promising therapy subjects patient's blood to Protein A (taken from the cell walls of a bacterium). When the blood is returned to breast cancer patients, their well-advanced tumors shrink by some 33 to 79 percent.

The process which somehow activates the patient's own immune system to destroy cancer cells was reported in November of 1981 by physicians at the Baylor College of Medicine in Houston. At that time it had shown benefits to three of five women. It definitely is not a cure, but the small experimental study received massive publicity because it opened "a new biological era" in treatment. Research will continue in this area and may yet lead to other and better procedures for shrinking tumors.

Many new drugs under investigation may play important roles in the future control of cancer. Interferon, a protein produced in minuscule amounts by the cells of the body, helps the body fight viruses ranging from chicken pox to the common cold. Early studies show interferon benefits one quarter of breast cancer patients, but the benefits are not long lasting. However, patients have been tested only with a relatively impure, expensive form of interferon. Newer and purer forms that may give more effective results are being produced, but it's too soon to tell how good they will be. Interferon is only one of the many new drugs constantly being analyzed with hopes of improving treatment.

Dozens of universities and cancer centers are experimenting with heat as another way to treat cancer. Heat therapy, called hyperthermia, is based on evidence that cancer cells don't like high temperatures. Normal cells don't either, but cancer cells are believed to be more sensitive because they have poor blood circulation and can't distribute the heat as well to other areas. In some experimental programs, heat-generating radiowaves are directed at deep-seated tumors that have not responded to conventional treatments. Other centers are removing blood from patients, heating it, then replacing it, either throughout the entire body or only at the specific tumor area. Many problems must be worked out before hyperthermia will be a routine treatment, but some believe it will enhance the impact of chemotherapy and radiation. For example, there is evidence that heat makes cancer cells more sensitive to radiation. It may help by shrinking the tumor or activating the immune system to do a better job of attacking cancer cells. Some researchers predict that the future may see certain tumors treated only by heat therapy.

Another extremely important direction is that of identifying those women most likely to get breast cancer. In 1980, scientists from several universities, including the University of California at Berkeley, reported that a common gene exists among women from extremely high-risk families in which as many as 50 percent of all immediate relatives get breast cancer. A gene is the tiny hereditary unit that controls day-by-day functioning of cells. In this case it seems to influence the cells' susceptibility to breast cancer. Blood tests can determine which members of these unusually high-risk families carry this gene. The experiments are not yet beneficial for most women, but if scientists can understand what causes the disease to develop in this select group they may understand how it evolves in others. Since this gene exists, it's also possible that other breast cancer susceptibility genes can be found. If these could be identified, women could be screened, with the high-risk group being closely followed for the earliest sign of disease. They could be counseled about avoiding environmental cancer-causing agents and other risk factors, like high-fat diets, which might increase their odds of activating potential cancer.

Chemoprevention, a brand new direction, applies chemicals to patients at high risk of developing cancer in the hope that the drugs will prevent or reverse premalignant disease. For example, retinoids, synthetic forms of vitamin A, have been shown to prevent or reverse premalignant disease in cells in test tubes and in some laboratory animals. High natural doses of the vitamin can be toxic, but the laboratory-produced forms are not dangerous. In one clinical trial, the substance is being applied to abnormal, but not yet cancerous, cervical tissue. It's being used for persons who are at extremely high risk of developing skin cancer. Similar experiments are being considered with retinoids for the prevention of breast cancer. Clinical trials under way in Europe are evaluating whether progesterone applied through the skin of the breast may prevent or limit long-term breast cancer.

Many believe that most cancers are caused by environmental agents. Research at the University of California at San Francisco is trying to determine which agents from inside and outside the body reach the breast and what their role is in causing breast disease or breast cancer. Studies of breast fluid have determined that nicotine from cigarettes, caffeine from coffee and tea, a chemotherapeutic agent, Thiotepa, and a cholesterollike product, all known to cause mutations and cancer in animals or bacteria, gain rapid access to the breast. But the questions remain: Do they do anything when they reach the breast? If so, what and how? One theory holds that women with certain genes may have more difficulty detoxifying these agents than others. It's only a guess now, but there may be answers as researchers learn more about human genetics and what environmental factors are linked to a higher incidence of breast cancer in women.

And when considering new directions, it is important to look at the contributions women are continuing to make toward their own treatment. A comment from one forty-year-old woman typifies the new direction: "Twenty years ago, I didn't know I could work with my doctor to make informed decisions about my own health. Today, I can research health issues and diseases and discuss them with my friends. I can read in the newspaper about subjects we didn't even talk about two decades ago."

Today's woman is demanding to be educated and informed about her medical care and is able to discuss medical options with her physician.

As one health advocate told me, "You get what you expect from the medical system." There is solid evidence that women are beginning to expect more—both from their doctors and from themselves.

How to Examine Your Breasts

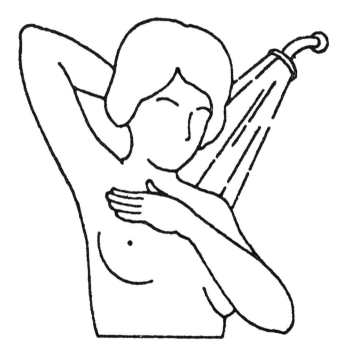

Step 1. In the shower

Examine your breasts during bath or shower; hands glide easier over wet skin. Fingers flat, move gently over every part of each breast. Use right hand to examine left breast, left hand for right breast. Check for any lump, hard knot, or thickening.

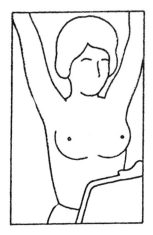 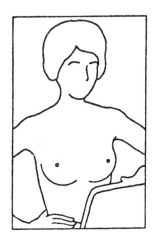

Step 2. Before a mirror

Inspect your breasts with arms at your sides. Next, raise your arms high overhead. Look for any changes in contour of each breast, a swelling, dimpling of skin, or changes in the nipple. Then, rest palms on hips and press down firmly to flex your chest muscles. Left and right breast will not exactly match—few women's do.

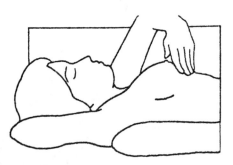

Step 3. Lying down

To examine your right breast, put a pillow or folded towel under your right shoulder. Place right hand behind your head—this distributes breast tissue more evenly on the chest. With left hand, fingers flat, press gently in small circular motions around an imaginary clock face.

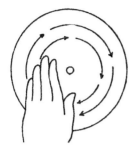 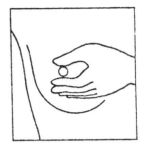

Begin at outermost top of your right breast for 12 o'clock, then move to 1 o'clock, and so on around the circle back to 12. A ridge of firm tissue in the lower curve of each breast is normal. Then move in an inch, toward the nipple, keep circling to examine every part of your breast, including nipple. This requires at least three more circles. Now slowly repeat procedure on your left breast with a pillow under your left shoulder and left hand behind head. Notice how your breast structure feels.

Finally, squeeze the nipple of each breast gently between thumb and index finger. Any discharge, clear or bloody, should be reported to your doctor immediately.

Information and pictures used with permission from the American Cancer Society, Inc.

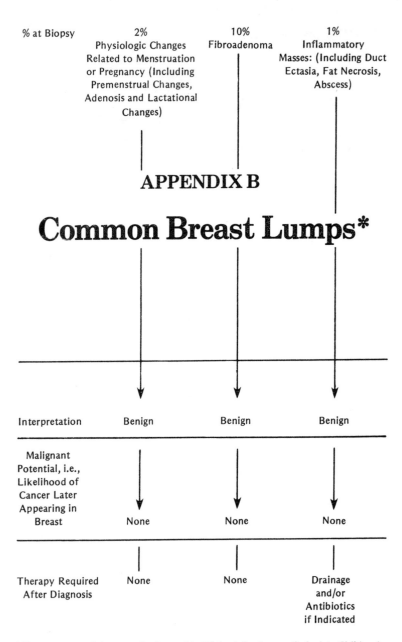

% at Biopsy	2% Physiologic Changes Related to Menstruation or Pregnancy (Including Premenstrual Changes, Adenosis and Lactational Changes)	10% Fibroadenoma	1% Inflammatory Masses: (Including Duct Ectasia, Fat Necrosis, Abscess)

APPENDIX B

Common Breast Lumps*

Interpretation	Benign	Benign	Benign
Malignant Potential, i.e., Likelihood of Cancer Later Appearing in Breast	None	None	None
Therapy Required After Diagnosis	None	None	Drainage and/or Antibiotics if Indicated

*Figure prepared in consultation with Michael Lagios, pathologist, Children's Hospital, San Francisco

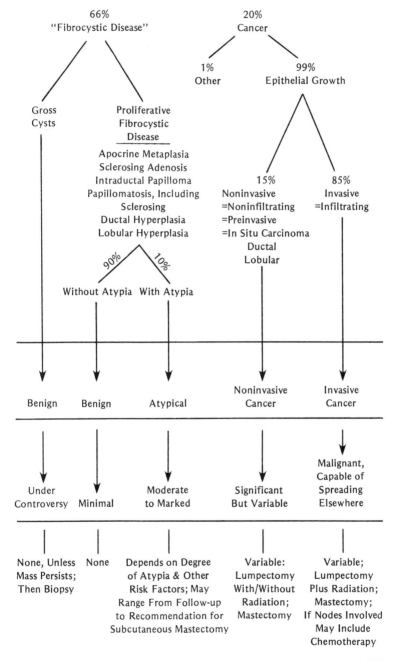

66%
"Fibrocystic Disease"

20%
Cancer

1%
Other

99%
Epithelial Growth

Gross
Cysts

Proliferative
Fibrocystic
Disease

Apocrine Metaplasia
Sclerosing Adenosis
Intraductal Papilloma
Papillomatosis, Including
Sclerosing
Ductal Hyperplasia
Lobular Hyperplasia

15%
Noninvasive
=Noninfiltrating
=Preinvasive
=In Situ Carcinoma
Ductal
Lobular

85%
Invasive
=Infiltrating

90%   10%

Without Atypia   With Atypia

Benign   Benign   Atypical

Noninvasive
Cancer

Invasive
Cancer

Malignant,
Capable of
Spreading
Elsewhere

Under
Controversy   Minimal

Moderate
to Marked

Significant
But Variable

None, Unless   None
Mass Persists;
Then Biopsy

Depends on Degree
of Atypia & Other
Risk Factors; May
Range From Follow-up
to Recommendation for
Subcutaneous Mastectomy

Variable:
Lumpectomy
With/Without
Radiation;
Mastectomy

Variable;
Lumpectomy
Plus Radiation;
Mastectomy;
If Nodes Involved
May Include
Chemotherapy

197

Definitions of Types of Surgery

Axillary Dissection: An incision made under the armpit to remove a variable number of lymph nodes. Experts on the 1979 Consensus panel agreed this should be combined with a Total Mastectomy for standard treatment of early breast cancer.

Incisional Biopsy: Surgical removal of a portion of tissue to be examined

Excisional Biopsy: Total surgical removal of tissue to be examined

Lumpectomy or Tylectomy: Removal of tumor plus a wedge of surrounding tissue

Quadrant Mastectomy: Removal of one quarter of the breast

Partial Mastectomy: Removal of part of breast

Wedge Resection: Removal of segment of breast, usually about one quarter

Segmental Resection: Removal of segment of breast

Hemimastectomy: Removal of one half of breast

Simple, Total, or
Complete Mastectomy: Removal of the breast. Most, if not all chest muscles left intact

Modified Radical
Mastectomy: Amputation of the breast and lymph nodes in the armpit. Chest muscles usually left intact. Variation: removal of the pectoralis minor muscle

Radical Mastectomy,
sometimes called the

Halsted Mastectomy: Amputation of the breast, the fat and skin surrounding the breast, the two muscles on front of the chest, and the fat and lymph nodes in the armpit

Extended Radical

Mastectomy: Radical plus removal of internal mammary nodes under the chest bone and possibly some of the rib cage

Types of Plastic Surgery

Augmentation Mammaplasty: Breast enlargement, usually by making a small incision in the fold beneath the breast and inserting an implant between the breast and chest muscle. Scar is hidden by the overhanging breast. Can be done as an outpatient under a local anesthetic.

Mastopexy: Breast lift to remove sagging of skin caused by pregnancy, weight loss, aging, and the pull of gravity. Same scars as from breast reduction, although in this case only skin, little internal breast tissue, is disturbed. Can be done as an outpatient under a local anesthetic in most cases.

Reconstruction Mammaplasty: Breast reconstruction procedure used by plastic surgeons to create a natural-looking breast shape after a breast has been removed to treat cancer.

Reduction Mammaplasty: Breast reduction. Usually surgeon makes a circular incision around the areola, down the underside of the breast and under the breast fold, the crease where breast meets the chest wall. Results in an "inverted T" or "anchor scar." Process almost always involves moving the nipple to a higher position on the breast. Almost always done in a hospital under general anesthetic. Variation: surgeon makes an incision around the nipple and across outside of breast.

Subcutaneous Mastectomy: Approximately 85 percent of tissue removed from breast, replaced with silicone pad insert. Nipple and skin left intact.

Common Drugs and Their Possible Side Effects in the Treatment of Breast Cancer

Adriamycin: Injected into a vein. Possible side effects include mild nausea and vomiting, which may occur within hours following the injection. For a few days following the injection, you may feel extremely tired. Painful sores in your mouth and or diarrhea may develop. Marked hair loss is common, but is usually reversible after therapy is stopped. Adriamycin may turn your urine red for a few hours after the injection, but this is related to the color of the drug and is nothing to be concerned about. Adriamycin may cause infertility or damage to an unborn fetus. Increased susceptibility to infection may occur. It may affect the heart muscle. If you should experience any chest pain, breathlessness, or irregular heart action, phone your physician.

Cyclophosphamide: Injected into a vein or given in pill form. The most common effects are loss of appetite, nausea, vomiting, and hair loss. Bladder irritation with bleeding can occur. Can cause infertility.

Methotrexate: Injected into a vein or given in pill form. Nausea and vomiting may occur within a few hours of administration. For a few days following administration, you may experience watery and itchy eyes, a runny nose, and loss of balance. You may be more susceptible to infection. Do not take any aspirin or aspirin-containing products while taking this drug.

5-Fluorouracil (5-FU): Injected into a vein. Nausea and vomiting are common, usually within a few hours following the injection. You may experience loss of balance and dizziness for a few days following the injection. Sores in your mouth and/or diarrhea may develop. Hair loss can occur.

Vincristine: Injected into a vein. Numbness and tingling of the feet and fingers along with pain in the throat or jaw are common. Less common are weakness of the hands and feet, loss of balance and reflexes, and a decrease in muscle size. Hair loss may occur. Vincristine may cause constipation, infertility, and harm an unborn fetus. Do not receive any immunizations without first notifying your physician.

Prednisone: Given in pill form. Side effects, usually associated with long-term therapy, may include muscle weakness, weight gain, salt retention, ankle swelling, and, rarely, mood changes. Peptic ulcers may become worse. This drug may cause infertility and damage an unborn fetus. Do not receive any immunizations without first consulting your physician.

Possible Side Effects of Hormones Given for Breast Cancer Therapy

Antiestrogen

Tamoxifen: Given in pill form. Common side effects include nausea, possible hot flashes, and breast enlargement.

Estrogens (female sex hormones)

Diethylstilbestrol: Given in pill form. Common side effects include nausea, vomiting, and cramps. Occasional side effects include fluid retention, lowered blood calcium, uterine bleeding.

Ethinyl estradiol: Given in pill form. Occasional side effects include fluid retention, lowered blood calcium, uterine bleeding.

Progestogens

Megestrol acetate: Given in pill form. No reported side effects.

Medroxyprogesterone acetate: Given in pill form or injected into a muscle. No major toxic side effects.

Hydroxyprogesterone: Injected into a muscle. No major toxic side effects.

Androgens (male sex hormones)

Fluoxymesterone: Given in pill form. Occasional side effects include fluid retention, masculinization (increased body hair and sex drive), jaundice, lowered blood calcium.

Cancer Information Service Telephone Numbers

The Cancer Information Service (CIS) is a toll-free telephone service established by the National Cancer Institute to answer the public's questions about cancer. The service provides information on resources and studies going on in your own area and can provide up-to-date information on research and treatment options. Numbers are effective as of March 1981.

For information call:

Alabama
1-800-292-6201
Alaska
1-800-638-6070
California
From Area Codes
(213), (714) and (805):
1-800-252-9066
Connecticut
1-800-922-0824
Delaware
1-800-523-3586
District of Columbia
(Includes suburbs in
Maryland and
Virginia)
636-5700
Florida
1-800-432-5953
Georgia
1-800-327-7332
Hawaii
Oahu: 524-1234

Neighbor Islands:
Ask operator for
Enterprise 6702
Illinois
800-972-0586
Kentucky
800-432-9321
Maine
1-800-225-7034
Maryland
800-492-1444
Massachusetts
1-800-952-7420
Minnesota
1-800-582-5262
New Hampshire
1-800-225-7034
New Jersey
(Northern)
800-223-1000
New Jersey
(Southern)
800-523-3586

New York State
1-800-462-7255
New York City
(212) 794-7982
North Carolina
1-800-672-0943
North Dakota
1-800-328-5188
Ohio
1-800-282-6522
Pennsylvania
1-800-822-3963
South Dakota
1-800-328-5188
Texas
1-800-392-2040
Vermont
1-800-225-7034
Washington
1-800-552-7212
Wisconsin
1-800-362-8038

All other areas 800-638-6694

Cancer Centers

Comprehensive Cancer Centers

Comprehensive Cancer Centers are specially designated institutes of excellence funded in part by the National Cancer Institute. The centers conduct a broad range of scientific research and develop and demonstrate methods of cancer prevention, diagnosis, treatment, and rehabilitation. Patients accepted for treatment are offered complete cancer care by physicians working in the centers. Comprehensive Cancer Centers are noted in the listing of cancer centers with a single asterisk(*).

Community-based Cancer Control Programs

The National Cancer Institute funds several Community-based Cancer Control Programs. Creation of these programs was based on the conviction that cancer patients can be most effectively and efficiently cared for if local resources are combined in a cooperative effort. Maximum use is made of community physicians, clinics, hospitals, and other local resources to prevent, detect, diagnose, treat, rehabilitate, and provide continuing care for cancer patients. Community-Based Cancer Control Programs are noted in the listing of cancer centers with two asterisks(**).

Other institutions around the country also specialize in services for the cancer patient. If a patient does not live near any of the cancer centers listed, she should call the nearest medical school or Cancer Information Service. A state-by-state listing of medical institutions offering care to breast cancer and other cancer patients follows:*

*Information supplied by National Cancer Institute.

ALABAMA

*Comprehensive Cancer Center
University of Alabama in Birmingham
University of Alabama Hospitals
and Clinics
619 South 19th Street
Birmingham, AL 35233
(205) 934-2651

CALIFORNIA

**Community Cancer Control
Los Angeles
5800 Wilshire Boulevard
Los Angeles, CA 90036
(213) 938-2608

*Los Angeles County University of
Southern California
Comprehensive Cancer Center
School of Medicine
2025 Zonal Avenue
Los Angeles, CA 90033
(213) 226-2008

Mt. Zion Hospital
1600 Divisadero
San Francisco, CA 94119
(415) 567-6600

Northern California Cancer Program
1801 Page Mill Road
Suite 190
Palo Alto, CA 94304
(415) 497-5353

Stanford University Medical Center
Stanford, CA 94305
(415) 497-7313
(415) 497-5055

*UCLA Comprehensive Cancer Center
UCLA School of Medicine
924 Westwood Boulevard
Suite 650
Los Angeles, CA 90024
(213) 825-1532
(213) 825-5268

West Coast Cancer Foundation
50 Francisco Street
Suite 200
San Francisco, CA 94133
(415) 563-5213

CONNECTICUT

*Yale University Comprehensive
Cancer Center

333 Cedar Street
New Haven, CT 06510
(203) 432-4122

DELAWARE

The Wilmington Medical Center
14th and Washington Streets
Wilmington, DE 19899
(302) 428-1212

DISTRICT OF COLUMBIA

*Georgetown University/Howard
University
Comprehensive Cancer Center
● Georgetown University
Medical Center
Lombardi Cancer Research
Center
3800 Reservoir Road, N.W.
Washington, DC 20007
(202) 625-7066

● Howard University Cancer
Research Center
Howard University Hospital
Department of Oncology
2041 Georgia Avenue, N.W.
Washington, DC 20007
(202) 625-7066

FLORIDA

*Comprehensive Cancer Center for
the State of Florida
University of Miami School of
Medicine/Jackson Memorial
Medical Center
Centre House, Roof Garden
1400 Northwest 10th Avenue
Miami, FL 33136
(305) 547-6758

GEORGIA

Emory University Cancer Center
Emory University Hospital
Room 606F
Atlanta, GA 30322
(404) 329-7016

HAWAII

**Cancer Center of Hawaii
University of Hawaii at Manoa
1997 East-West Road
Honolulu, HI 90822
(808) 948-7246

IDAHO
Mountain States Tumor Institute
151 East Bannock
Boise, ID 83702
(208) 386-2711

ILLINOIS
*Illinois Cancer Council
37 South Wabash Avenue
Chicago, IL 60603
(312) 346-9813

- Northwestern University
  Cancer Center
  Ward Memorial Building
  303 East Chicago Avenue
  Chicago, IL 60611
  (312) 649-8674

- Rush Cancer Center
  1725 West Harrison
  Chicago, IL 60612
  (312) 947-6386

- University of Chicago Cancer
  Research Center
  905 East 59th Street
  Chicago, IL 60637
  (312) 947-6386

KANSAS
Mid-America Cancer Center Program
The University of Kansas
  Medical Center
College of Health Sciences
  and Hospital
Rainbow Boulevard at 39th
Kansas City, KS 66103
(913) 588-5700

KENTUCKY
University of Louisville
Health Sciences Center
Walnut and Preston Streets
Louisville, KY 40202
(502) 582-2211

MARYLAND
*Johns Hopkins Oncology Center
601 North Broadway
Baltimore, MD 21205
(301) 955-8822

MASSACHUSETTS
Boston University Cancer
  Research Center
80 East Concord Street
Boston, MA 02118
(617) 247-6075

Cox Cancer Center
Massachusetts General Hospital
100 Blossom Street
Boston, MA 02114
(617) 726-8660

New England Medical Center Hospital
171 Harrison Avenue
Boston, MA 02111
(617) 482-2800, Ext. 2672

*Sidney Farber Cancer Institute
44 Binney Street
Boston, MA 02115
(617) 739-1100, Ext. 3140 or 3149

MICHIGAN
*Michigan Cancer Foundation/
  Wayne State University
110 East Warren Avenue
Detroit, MI 48201
(313) 833-0710

MINNESOTA
*Mayo Comprehensive
  Cancer Center
200 First Street, S.W.
Rochester, MN 55901
(507) 282-2511

MISSOURI
Missouri Cancer Programs, Inc.
115 Business Loop 70 West
Columbia, MO 65201
(314) 449-3445

NEW HAMPSHIRE
Norris Cotton Center of the
Dartmouth-Hitchcock Medical Center
Hanover, NH 03755
(603) 643-4000, Ext. 2441

NEW MEXICO
**New Mexico Cancer Research
  Treatment Center

900 Camino de Salud, N.E.
Albuquerque, NM 87131
(505) 277-3631

NEW YORK

Albany Medical College of
  Union University
Albany Medical Center Hospital
New Scotland Avenue
Albany, NY 12208
(215) 445-5307

Albert Einstein College of Medicine
1300 Morris Park Avenue
Bronx, NY 10461
(212) 430-2302
(212) 792-2233

Columbia University Cancer
  Research Center
College of Physicians and Surgeons
701 West 168th Street
New York, NY 10032
(212) 694-3807
(212) 694-4138

Hospital for Joint Diseases and
  Medical Center
1919 Madison Avenue
New York, NY 10035
(212) 876-7222

**Long Island Cancer Council
560 Broad Hollow Road
Melville, NY 11746
(516) 249-2688

*Memorial Sloan-Kettering
  Cancer Center
1275 York Avenue
New York, NY 10021
(212) 794-7000

Mt. Sinai Hospital
Fifth Avenue and 100th Street
New York, NY 10003
(212) 650-6500

New York University Medical Center
Department of Medicine
550 First Avenue
New York, NY 10016
(212) 679-3200

*Roswell Park Memorial Institute

666 Elm Street
Buffalo, NY 14263
(716) 845-5770

State University of New York
Downstate Medical Center
450 Clarkson Avenue
Brooklyn, NY 11203
(212) 270-1000

The Strang Clinic
55 East 34th Street
New York, NY 10016
(212) 683-1000

University of Rochester Cancer Center
601 Elmwood Avenue
Rochester, NY 14642
(716) 275-4865

NORTH CAROLINA

*Duke University Medical Center
Comprehensive Cancer Center
200 Atlas Street
Durham, NC 27705
(919) 684-8111

Cancer Research Center
University of North Carolina
P.O. Box 3
Swing Building 217H
Chapel Hill, NC 27514
(919) 966-1183
(919) 966-3036

Bowman Gray School of Medicine
300 South Hawthorne Road
Winston-Salem, NC 27103
(919) 727-4464

OHIO

*The Ohio State University Compre-
  hensive Cancer Center
1580 Cannon Drive
Columbus, OH 43210
(614) 422-5022

Cleveland Clinic Cancer Center
9500 Euclid Avenue
Cleveland, OH 44106
(216) 444-2445

OKLAHOMA

Oklahoma Cancer Center

University of Oklahoma
Health Services Center
P.O. Box 26901
Oklahoma City, OK 73190
(405) 271-4485

PENNSYLVANIA

*Fox Chase/University of
Pennsylvania Comprehensive
Cancer Center
Fox Chase Cancer Center
7701 Burholme Avenue
Fox Chase
Philadelphia, PA 19111
(215) 342-1000

Jefferson Medical College
11th and Walnut Streets
Philadelphia, PA 19107
(215) 928-6000

PUERTO RICO

Puerto Rico Cancer Center
University of Puerto Rico
Medical Sciences Campus
G.P.O. Box 5067
San Juan, PR 00936
(809) 763-2443
(809) 765-2363

RHODE ISLAND

Roger Williams General Hospital
825 Chalkstone Avenue
Providence, RI 02908
(401) 456-2070

**Rhode Island Cancer
Control Program
345 Blackstone Boulevard
Providence, RI 02906
(401) 351-0500

TENNESSEE

Memphis Regional Cancer Center
800 Madison Avenue
Memphis, TN 38163
(901) 528-5739

TEXAS

*The University of Texas System
Cancer Center
M.D. Anderson Hospital and
Tumor Institute
6723 Bertner Avenue

Houston, TX 77030
(713) 792-3000

● University of Texas Health
Sciences Center
5323 Harry Hines Boulevard
Dallas, TX 75235
(214) 688-2166

● The University of Texas
Medical Branch
Administration Building
Suite 645
Galveston, TX 77550
(713) 765-1902

VERMONT

Vermont Regional Cancer Center
One South Prospect Street
Burlington, VT 05405
(802) 656-4414

VIRGINIA

MCV/VCU Cancer Center
P.O. Box 37 MCV Station
Medical College of Virginia
Virginia Commonwealth University
Richmond, VA 23298
(804) 770-7682
(804) 770-7476

WASHINGTON

*Fred Hutchinson Cancer
Research Center
1124 Columbia Street
Seattle, WA 98104
(206) 292-2930

WISCONSIN

Marshfield Clinic
1000 North Oak Avenue
Marshfield, WI 54449
(715) 387-5511

*The University of Wisconsin Clinical
Cancer Center
600 Highland Avenue
Madison, WI 53792
(608) 262-0046

Medical College of Wisconsin
1700 West Wisconsin Avenue
Milwaukee, WI 53233
(414) 344-7100, Ext. 374

Additional Sources of Information

American Cancer Society

Consists of fifty-eight chartered divisions and nearly 3,000 local units set up to offer basic service programs to cancer patients and their families. May loan sick room equipment and provide counseling and information. Can put you in contact with Reach to Recovery volunteer. You can reach local units in most areas by looking in the white pages under American Cancer Society. National Office: American Cancer Society, 777 Third Avenue, New York, NY 10017.

Breast Cancer Advisory Center:

Director: Rose Kushner
11426 Rockville Pike
Suite 406
Rockville, MD 20850

Volunteer group can mail information sheets and answer questions about all aspects of cancer diagnoses and treatment.

Breast Reconstruction:

American Society of Plastic and Reconstructive Surgeons
233 E. Michigan Ave.
Suite 1900
Chicago, IL 60601
(312) 856-1818

Volunteer groups set up to provide accurate, current information about breast reconstruction and arrange for you to talk to another woman who has had the surgery. (Some operate under auspices of their area American Cancer Society divisions.)

AFTER

Ask A Friend to Explain Reconstruction
1378 Third Ave.
New York, NY 10021
(212) 472-0040

AWEAR

A Woman Educating About Reconstruction
1-800-552-7996 (toll-free); in Richmond, Virginia, area call 359-0208

IMAGES AND OPTIONS

In San Francisco Bay Area
(415) 522-2924

RENU

Reconstruction Education for National Understanding
Cleveland has a twenty-four-hour answering service (216) 444-2900
Washington, DC (202) 483-2600

ENCORE
YWCA

For postoperative breast cancer patients. Exercise plan (usually includes some swimming) plus discussion group. Call your local YWCA branch to see if it exists in your area, or write ENCORE National Board YWCA, 600 Lexington Ave., New York, NY 10022.

Make Today Count, Inc.
P.O. Box 303
Burlington, IA 52601 (319) 753-6521

Provides psychological assistance to patients with advanced cancer and to their families. Group meetings, home visit programs, newsletters. Founded by Orville E. Kelly, a cancer patient. Over 300 chapters located throughout the country. Look in local directory or write to above address.

National Hospice Organization
1311A Dolley Madison Boulevard
McLean, VA 22101
(703) 356-6770

The hospice movement offers supportive care for terminally ill patients. The program is concerned with the quality of care that patients receive when medicine can no longer offer hope of cure. More than 500 programs now exist in the United States. The national office can tell you if services exist in your area.

A Breast Cancer Patient's Options and Rights*

- to receive a simple and clear diagnosis of her condition.
- to receive all available diagnostic procedures and a complete work-up prior to surgery.
- to have the consent form clearly explained to her before she signs it.
- to have the biopsy performed first (under local anesthesia), including the right to see the pathologist's report and have it explained to her. Surgery may be performed at a later date.
- to be aware that for certain patients the future option of reconstructive plastic surgery exists and to have the surgeon take that option into consideration.
- to receive consideration from the surgeon and other medical personnel for the physical and emotional trauma she is undergoing.
- to receive an explanation of any viable alternative treatments—including biopsy with radiation therapy as primary treatment, chemotherapy, immunotherapy, mastectomy, etc., risks, disadvantages, and advantages of each treatment.
- to receive a satisfying explanation as to why the surgeon has decided on a particular surgical procedure rather than a less mutilating one.
- to be referred to a therapist for physical or psychiatric therapy following surgery.

*Prepared by Women for Women, a nonprofit organization formed on the West Coast, dealing with problems associated with breast cancer.

- to receive competent follow-up care after surgery and to know who is going to be responsible for that care.
- to be referred to a support group for information and assistance with her personal concerns.
- to be always treated as an adult.

The Living Will

TO MY FAMILY, MY PHYSICIAN, MY CLERGYMAN,
MY LAWYER—

If the time comes when I can no longer take part in decisions for my own future, let this statement stand as the testament of my wishes:

If there is no reasonable expectation of my recovery, from physical or mental disability, I＿＿＿＿＿＿＿＿＿＿＿＿＿＿, request that I be allowed to die and not be kept alive by artificial means or heroic measures. Death is as much a reality as birth, growth, maturity, and old age—it is the one certainty. I do not fear death as much as I fear indignity, deterioration, dependence, and hopeless pain. I ask that medication be mercifully administered to me for terminal suffering even if it hastens the moment of death.

This request is made after careful consideration. Although this document is not legally binding, you who care for me will, I hope, feel morally bound to follow its mandate. I recognize that this places a heavy burden of responsibility upon you, and it is with the intention of sharing that responsibility and of mitigating any feelings of guilt that this statement is made.

Signer: ＿＿＿＿＿＿＿＿＿＿＿＿＿

Date: ＿＿＿＿＿＿

WITNESSED by:

_____

_____

Bibliography

The following are the major references and sources I used in writing this book. Articles are listed under the name of the first author. My most important source of information was the week-long 19th National Conference on Breast Cancer, March 9–13, 1981, Hotel Del Coronado, San Diego. The program was sponsored by the American College of Radiology and co-sponsored by the American Cancer Society, the College of American Pathologists, the Educational Foundation of Plastic and Reconstructive Surgeons, and the Society for the Study of Breast Disease.

Publications I referred to for almost every chapter include *The Breast Cancer Digest*, produced in 1979 by the National Cancer Institute's Office of Cancer Communication (Publication No. 80-1691); *The Breast*, edited by H. Stephen Gallager, Henry Patrick Leis, Jr., Reuven K. Snyderman, and Jerome A. Urban, published in 1978 by C. V. Mosby, St. Louis; *Cancer of the Breast*, edited by W. L. Donegan and J. S. Spratt, published in 1979 by W. B. Saunders, Philadelphia; *Diseases of the Breast* by C. D. Haagensen, 1971 edition, published by W. B. Saunders. Readers interested in more extensive discussion of topics may refer to any of these books as well as those listed in Selected Readings.

Chapter 2: A Lump: What Does It Mean?

Azzopardi, John G. *Problems In Breast Pathology*. W. B. Saunders, 1979.

Belson, Abby Avin. "Medical Update: Benign Breast Disorders." *Women's Day*, November 20, 1978.

Black, M. "Association of Atypical Characteristics of Benign Breast Lesions with Subsequent Risk of Breast Cancer." *Cancer* 29:338–343, 1972.

Black, Shirley Temple. "Don't Sit Home and Be Afraid." *McCall's*, February 1973, p. 82.

Bland, Kirby L. "Analysis of Breast Cancer Screening in Women Younger Than 50 Years." *JAMA*, March 13, 1981.

"The Breast Disease That Isn't Cancer." *Good Housekeeping,* August 1980, p. 210.

Donegan, William. "Diagnosis." Chapter 3 in *Cancer of the Breast,* ed. W. L. Donegan and J. S. Spratt. W. B. Saunders, 1979.

Gallup Organization. Women's Attitudes Regarding Breast Cancer. November 7, 1973.

Haagensen, C. D. "The Relationship of Gross Cystic Disease of the Breast and Carcinoma." *Ann. Surg.,* March 1977.

Haagensen, C. D. "The Technique of Excision of Benign Tumors of the Breast," Chapter 6 in *Diseases of the Breast.* W. B. Saunders, 1971.

Hunt, T. K. "Breast Biopsies on Outpatient Surgeries." *Surg. Gynecol. Obstet.* 141:591, 1975.

Lagios, Michael D. "Interpretations of Pathological Diagnosis in Breast Carcinoma." Chapter 3, in *Post-Mastectomy Reconstruction,* ed. T. D. Gant and L. O. Vasconez. Williams and Wilkens, Baltimore, 1981.

Leis, Henry Patrick, Jr. *The Diagnosis of Breast Cancer.* American Cancer Society, Professional Education Publication, 1977.

Leis, Henry Patrick, Jr. "Fibrocystic Disease of the Breast." *J. Reprod. Med.,* vol. 22, no. 6, June 1979.

Leis, Henry Patrick, Jr., "Nipple Discharge." *Am. J. Diagnost. Gyn. and Obstet.,* vol. 1, no. 1, Spring 1979.

McLean, Martha. *If You Find a Lump in Your Breast . . .* Bull Publishing, Palo Alto, 1980.

Minton, John P. "Caffeine, Cyclic Nucleotides and Breast Disease." *Surgery,* July 1979.

Minton, John P. "Clinical and Biochemical Studies on Methylxanthine-related Fibrocystic Breast Disease." *Surgery,* August 1981.

National Institutes of Health Consensus Development Conference Summary, *Steroid Receptors in Breast Cancer,* vol. 2, no. 6, n.d.

Page, D. L. "Relationship Between Component Parts of Fibrocystic Disease Complex and Breast Cancer." *J. Natl. Cancer Inst.,* vol. 61, no. 4, Oct. 1978.

Sartorius, O. "Cytologic Evaluation of Breast Fluid in the Detection of Breast Disease." *J. Natl. Cancer Inst.,* vol. 59, no. 4, Oct. 1977.

Sartorius, O. "Needle Aspiration for Cytologic Diagnosis of Benign and Malignant Breast Lesions," paper presented before American College of Surgeons, Palm Springs, CA, Jan. 1980.

Shingleton, W. "Breast Biopsy Techniques," paper presented at 19th National Conference on Breast Cancer, San Diego, CA, March 1981.

Special Report of the Working Group to Review the NCI-ACS Breast Cancer Detection Demonstration Projects. *J. Natl. Cancer Inst.* vol. 62, no. 3, 1979.

Sundaram, G. "A-tocopherol and Serum Lipoproteins." *Lipids,* vol. 16, no. 4, April 1981.

Tabar, Laszlo. "Screening for Breast Cancer: The Swedish Trial." *Radiology* 138:219–222, Jan. 1981.

Wellings, S. R. "An Atlas of Subgross Pathology of the Human Breast with Special Reference to Possible Precancerous Lesions. *J. Natl. Cancer Inst.*, vol. 55, 1975.

Chapter 3: Your Risk and What to Do About It

Black, M. "Family History and Oral Contraceptives." *Cancer* 46:2747, 1980.

Blot, W. J. "Changing Patterns of Breast Cancer Among American Women." *Am. J. Pub. Health*, vol. 7, no. 8, 1980.

Blot, W. J. "Geographic Patterns of Breast Cancer in the United States." *J. Natl. Cancer Inst.*, vol. 59, no. 5, November 1977.

"Breast Cancer, Some Trying Surgery as a Preventive." Los Angeles *Times*, Dec. 9, 1980.

"Breast Surgery Before Cancer." *Newsweek*, Dec. 1, 1980.

"Breast Type Doesn't Affect Cancer Risk, Study Finds." *Medical World News*, Nov. 12, 1979.

Buell, Philip. "Changing Incidence of Breast Cancer in Japanese-American Women." *J. Natl. Cancer Inst.*, vol. 51, no. 5, Nov. 1973.

Dowden, Richard V. "Total Mastectomy for Premalignant Disease with Immediate Reconstruction." Chapter 9 in *Post-Mastectomy Reconstruction*, ed. T. D. Gant and L. O. Vasconez, Williams and Wilkins, Baltimore, 1981.

"Epidemiology and Etiology of Breast Cancer." Special Report, *N. Engl. J. Med.*, Nov. 20, 1980.

"Estrogen Therapy and Breast Cancer." *Science News*, vol. 117, May 3, 1980.

Fasal, Elfriede. "Oral Contraceptives as Related to Cancer and Benign Lesions of the Breast." *J. Natl. Cancer Inst.* 55:767, 1975.

Gray, G. E. "Breast Cancer Incidence and Mortality Rates in Different Countries in Relation to Known Risk Factors and Dietary Practices." *Br. J. Cancer*, vol. 39, no. 1, 1979.

Hoffman, S. "Alternatives to the Subcutaneous Mastectomy." *Plast. Reconstr. Surg.*, August 1979.

Hoover, Robert. "Menopausal Estrogens and Breast Cancer. *N. Engl. J. Med.*, vol. 295, no. 8, Aug. 19, 1976.

"Incidence and Mortality in the United States." *J. Natl. Cancer Inst.*, Monograph 57, NIG No. 81-230, June 1981.

Kelly, Patricia T. "Familial Breast Cancer: New Data Show Lower Risks for Some Sisters and Daughters." *Your Patient and Cancer*, May 1981.

Kelly, Patricia T. "Refinements in Breast Cancer Risk Analysis." *Arch. Surg.*, vol. 116, March 1981.

Leis, Henry Patrick, Jr. "Epidemiology of Breast Cancer: Identification of the High-Risk Woman." In *The Breast*, ed. H. Stephen Gallager and Henry Patrick Leis, Jr. C. V. Mosby, 1978.

Leis, Henry Patrick, Jr. "Risk Factors for Breast Cancer: An Update." *Breast, Diseases of the Breast*, vol. 6, no. 4.

MacMahon, Brian. "Etiology of Human Breast Cancer: A Review." *J. Natl. Cancer Inst.*, vol. 50, no. 1, January 1973.

McConnell, Kenneth P. "The Relationship of Dietary Selenium and Breast Cancer," *J. Surg. Oncol.*, 15:67–70, 1980.

Miller, A. B. "Nutrition and Cancer." *Prev. Med.* 9:189, 1980.

Miller, A. B. "A Study of Diet and Breast Cancer." *Am. J. Epidemiol.*, vol. 107, no. 6, October-December 1980.

Peacock Earl. "Biological Basis for Management of Benign Disease of the Breast: The Case Against Subcutaneous Mastectomy." *Plast. Reconstr. Surg.*, January 1975.

Pennisi, Vincent. "Indications, Contraindications and Complications of Subcutaneous Mastectomy." Chapter 8 in *Post-Mastectomy Reconstruction*, ed. T. D. Gant and L. O. Vasconez, Williams and Wilkins, Baltimore, 1981.

Pennisi, Vincent. "The Prevention of Breast Cancer by the Subcutaneous Mastectomy." *Surg. Clin. North Am.*, vol. 57, no. 5, October 1977, p. 1023.

Petrakis, Nicholas. "Genetic Factors in the Etiology of Breast Cancer." *Cancer*, June supplement 39:2709, 1977.

Petrakis, Nicholas, Ernster, Virginia, and King, Mary-Claire. "The Epidemiology of Breast Cancer." In *Cancer Epidemiology and Prevention*, ed. D. Schottenfeld and J. Fraumeni, Jr., forthcoming.

Pike, M. C., "Oral Contraceptive Use and Early Abortion as Risk Factors for Breast Cancer in Young Women," *Br. J. Cancer*, Jan. 1981.

Ross, Ronald K. "A Case-Control Study of Menopausal Estrogen Therapy and Breast Cancer." *JAMA*, April 25, 1980.

Schwartz, Gordon F. "The Clinical Implications of Risk Factors in Breast Cancer," paper presented at 19th National Conference on Breast Cancer, San Diego, March 1981.

Soini, Irma. "Failure of Selective Screening for Breast Cancer by Combining Risk Factors." *Int. J. Cancer* 22:275–281, 1978.

Wynder, Ernest. "Dietary Factors Related to Breast Cancer." *Cancer*, 46:899, 1980.

Vorherr, Helmuth. *Breast Cancer Epidemiology, Endocrinology, Biochemistry and Pathology.* Urban and Schwarzenberg, Baltimore, 1980.

Chapter 4: Breast Cancer Psychology

Asken, Michael. "Psychoemotional Aspects of Mastectomy, A Review of Recent Literature." *Am. J. Psychiatry*, January 1975.

Ayalah, Daphna, and Weinstock, Isaac, J. *Breasts: Women Speak About Their Breasts and Their Lives.* Summit Books, New York, 1979. (I took some of the comments on women's feelings about their breasts from this book.)

Bard, Morton. *"Adaptation to Radical Mastectomy,"* The Psychological Impact of Cancer, American Cancer Society, Professional Education Publication.

Bird, Rose Elizabeth. "Coming to Terms with the Fear of Cancer." Los Angeles *Times*, July 17, 1980.

Brand, P. C., and van Keep, P. A. *Breast Cancer, Psycho-Social Aspects of Early Detection and Treatment.* University Park Press, Baltimore, 1978.

"Breast Cancer, A Measure of Progress in Public Understanding." Technical Report, National Institutes of Health, Pub. No. 81-2291, October 1980.

Goin, Marcia Kraft. "Midlife Reactions to Mastectomy and Subsequent Breast Reconstruction." *Arch. Gen. Psychiatry*, vol. 38, February 1981.

Greer, S. "Psychological Consequences of Cancer." *Practitioner*, Feb. 22, 1979.

Holland, Jimmie. "Psychologic Adaptation to Breast Cancer." *Cancer*, August 1980, p. 1045.

Jamison, Kay R. "Psychological Aspects of Mastectomy: I, The Woman's Perspective." *Am. J. Psychiatry*, April 1978.

Klein, Roberta. "A Crisis to Grow On." *Cancer*, December 1971.

Maguire, G. P. "Psychiatric Problems in the First Year After Mastectomy." *Br. Med. J.*, April 15, 1978.

Masters W., and Johnson, V. "The Great Breast Mystique." *Redbook*, November 1975.

May, H. J. "Psychosexual Sequelae to Mastectomy: Implications for Therapeutic and Rehabilitative Intervention." *J. Rehabil.*, January 1980.

Mendelson, Bryan. "The Psychological Basis for Breast Reconstruction Following Mastectomy." *Med. J. Aust.*, May 31, 1980.

Meyerowitz, Beth E. "The Impact of Mastectomy on the Lives of Women." *Professional Psychol.*, vol. 12, no. 1, February 1981.

Meyerowitz, Beth E. "Psychological Correlates of Breast Cancer and Its Treatments." *Psychol. Bull.*, vol. 87, no. 1, January 1980.

Morris, T. "Psychological and Social Adjustment to Mastectomy." *Cancer* 40: 2381, 1977.

"My Problem and How I Solved It. I Didn't Feel Like A Real Woman Any More." *Good Housekeeping*, September 1977. I gave the name "Lynn" to the woman who anonymously described her experience in this article.

Rollin, Betty. *First You Cry*. J. B. Lippincott, Philadelphia, 1976.

Schain, Wendy. "Sexual Dysfunctions in Cancer Patients." In V. DeVita and S. Rosenberg, *Principles and Practices in Oncology*. J. B. Lippincott, Philadelphia, 1981.

Schain, Wendy. "Sexual Functioning, Self-Esteem and Cancer Care." Chapter in Breast Cancer: Its Impact on the Patient, Family and Community; proceedings of 11th Annual San Francisco Cancer Symposium, vol. 11, *Frontiers of Radiation Therapy and Oncology*, ed. J. Vaeth, Basel, N.Y. Karger, 1976.

Silverman, Joel. "Psychological Aspects of Breast Cancer and Reconstructive Surgery." *Va. Med. Mon.*, 106, February 1979.

Wellish, David K. "Psychosocial Aspects of Mastectomy: II, The Man's Perspective." *Am. J. Psychiatry*, May 1978.

Wortman, Camille. "Interpersonal Relationships and Cancer: A Theoretical Analysis," *J. Soc. Issues*, vol. 35, no. 1, 1979.

Zilbergeld, Bernie. *Male Sexuality*. Bantam Books, 1978.

Chapter 5: Where Are We Today?

American College of Surgeons Commission on Cancer. *Final Report on Long-Term Patient Care Evaluation Study for Carcinoma of the Female Breast.* 1979.

Bonadonna, Gianni. "Combination Chemotherapy as an Adjuvant Treatment in Operable Breast Cancer." *N. Engl. J. Med.,* Feb. 19, 1976.

Bonadonna, Gianni. "Dose-effect of Adjuvant Chemotherapy in Breast Cancer." *N. Engl. J. Med.,* Jan. 1, 1981.

Brody, E. "War on Cancer," Status Report: Progress Is Slow, but Gains Real. *New York Times,* April 14, 1981.

Brody, Jane E. "Cancer Therapies Improve." *New York Times,* April 15, 1981.

"Breast Cancer: Fear and Facts." *Time,* Nov. 4, 1974.

Breast Cancer: A Measure of Progress in Public Understanding, NIH Technical Report, Pub. No. 81-2291, Oct. 1980.

Breast Cancer Resource Guide I. National Women's Health Network, Washington, D.C., 1980.

"Breast Cancer: The Retreat from Radical Surgery." *Consumer Reports.* Feb. 2, 1981.

Cancer in California. Reference Issue of the *American Cancer Society Volunteer,* vol. 27, no. 1, 1981.

"Cancer Treatment, Clinical Trials vs. Local Teams." *Medical World News,* Jan. 5, 1981.

Cooper, William A. "The History of the Radical Mastectomy." *Annals of Medical History,* 3rd series, vol. 3, pp. 36–54, 1941.

Crile, George, Jr. "Management of Breast Cancer: Limited Mastectomy." *JAMA,* Oct. 7, 1974.

DeVita, Vincent T., Jr. "Cancer Mortality: The Good News." In *Adjuvant Therapy of Cancer II,* ed. S. Jones and S. Salmon. Grune and Stratton, New York, 1979.

Farrow, Joseph J. "Antiquity of Breast Cancer." *Cancer,* December 1971.

Feldman, Joseph G. "Breast Self-Examination, Relationship to Stage of Breast Cancer at Diagnosis." *Cancer,* June 1981.

Fisher, Bernard. "The Contribution of Recent NSABP Clinical Trials of Primary Breast Cancer Therapy to an Understanding of Tumor Biology—An Overview of Findings. *Cancer,* August supplement, 1980.

Fisher, Bernard. "The Evolution of Breast Cancer Surgery: Past, Present, and Future." *Semin. Oncol.,* vol. 5, no. 4, p. 386, Dec. 1978.

Fisher, Bernard. "Laboratory and Clinical Research in Breast Cancer—A Personal Adventure: The David A. Karnofsky Memorial Lecture." *Cancer Res.,* vol. 40, November 1980.

Fox, Maurice S. "On the Diagnosis and Treatment of Breast Cancer." *JAMA,* Feb. 2, 1979.

Haagensen, C. D. "A Great Leap Backward in the Treatment of Carcinoma of the Breast." *JAMA*, May 21, 1973.

Halsted, William. *Surgical Papers by Wm. Stewart Halsted.* Johns Hopkins Press, Baltimore, 1924.

Henny, Jane E. "The Evolution of Primary Multimodality Treatment in Resectable Breast Cancer." *Cancer*, August supplement, 1980.

Hunt, Thomas K. "Trends in Management of Cancer of the Breast," paper presented at meeting of Breast Neoplasia, Epidemiology, Diagnosis, Treatment, and Reconstruction, Park City, Utah, March 7-14, 1981.

Kushner, Rose. *Breast Cancer, A Personal History and an Investigative Report.* Harcourt Brace Jovanovich, New York, 1975.

Leis, Henry Patrick, Jr. "Cancer Trends in Breast Cancer Surgery in the U.S. and Canada." *Int. Surg.*, 65:3, 1980.

Lewison, Edward F. "Breast Cancer Surgery from Halsted to 1972." *Proc. Nat. Cancer Conf.* 7:275, 1973.

Lewison, Edward F. "Changing Concepts in Breast Cancer." *Cancer* 46:859-864, 1980.

McGehee, Harvey A. "Early Contributions to the Surgery of Cancer." *Johns Hopkins Med. J.*, December 1974.

Mansfield, Carl N. *Early Breast Cancer: Its History and Results of Treatment, Experimental Biology and Medicine*, vol. 5. Karger, 1976.

Public Health Reports. "Women and Health, United States." September-October 1980.

Morra, Marion, and Pots, Eve. *Choices: Realistic Alternatives in Cancer Treatment.* Avon, 1980.

National Institutes of Health Consensus Development Conference Summary, *The Treatment of Primary Cancer: Management of Local Disease*, vol. 2, no. 5, n.d.

Personal Communication. Harold Ellis, Professor of Surgery, Westminster Medical School, June 15, 1981.

Pollack, Earl. "Trends in Cancer Incidence and Mortality in the U.S., 1969–1976" *J. Natl. Cancer Inst.*, no. 5, 1980.

Roach, Marjorie. Testimony presented to the Massachusetts Legislature in support of Patient's Rights Bill No. 393, February 1979.

Shimkin, Michael. *Contrary to Nature.* Department of Health, Education, and Welfare, Government Printing Office, 1977.

Stehlin, J. S. "Treatment of Carcinoma of the Breast." *Surg. Gynecol. Obstet.*, December 1979.

Veronesi, Umberto. "Comparing Radical Mastectomy with Quadrantectomy, Axillary Dissection and Radiotherapy in Patients with Small Cancers of the Breast." *New Engl. J. Med.*, July 2, 1981.

Chapter 6: It's Cancer—Now What Happens?

Bedwani, Ramez. "Management and Survival of Female Patients with 'Minimal' Breast Cancer." *Cancer* 47:2769–2778, 1981.

Campion, Rosamond. "Five Years Later: No Regrets." *McCall's,* June 1976.

Cancer Patient Survival Experience, Trends in Survival 1960–63 to 1970–73. U.S. Department of Health and Human Services, NIH Pub. No. 80-2148, June 1980.

Carbonne Paul P. "Medical Treatment for Advanced Breast Cancer." *Sem. Oncol.,* vol. 5, no. 4, December 1978.

Carter, Stephen K. *Chemotherapy of Cancer.* John Wiley, 1981.

Curletti, Eugene. "In Situ, Lobular Carcinoma of the Breast." *Arch. Surg.,* March 1981.

Dietz, J. Herbert. *Rehabilitation of the Cancer Patient.* Professional Education Publication, American Cancer Society.

Donegan, William L. "Mammary Carcinoma and Pregnancy." Chapter 13 in *Cancer of the Breast,* ed. W. L. Donegan and J. S. Spratt. W. B. Saunders, 1979.

Dunphy, J. Englebert. Annual Discourse; on caring for the patient with cancer, *Cancer, a Manual for Practitioners,* Fifth Edition. American Cancer Society, Massachusetts Division, 1978.

"Final Word on Disputed Mastectomies." *Science,* Nov. 17, 1978.

Fisher, Bernard. "Pathological Findings from the NSABP." *Cancer* 46:908–918, 1980.

Haskell, Charles M. "Breast Cancer." Chapter 7 in *Cancer Treatment,* ed. Charles M. Haskell, W. B. Saunders Company, 1980.

Henderson, Craig. "Cancer of the Breast, the Past Decade." *New Engl. J. Med.,* Jan. 3, 1980.

Hunt, T. K. "Surgical Management of Breast Cancer," paper presented at meeting of Breast Neoplasia, Epidemiology, Diagnosis, Treatment, and Reconstruction, Park City, Utah, March 7–14, 1981.

Hutter, Robert V. "The Influence of Pathological Factors on Breast Cancer Management." *Cancer,* August supplement, 1980.

Jones, Stephen E. "Combination Chemotherapy for Advanced Breast Cancer." Monograph prepared for Adria Laboratories.

Kübler-Ross, Elisabeth. *On Death and Dying.* MacMillan, 1969.

Lagios, Michael. "Interpretation of Pathological Diagnosis in Breast Carcinoma." Chapter 3 in *Post-Mastectomy Reconstruction,* ed. T. D. Gant and L. O. Vas-Conez. Williams and Wilkins, 1981.

Manual for Staging of Cancer. American Joint Committee for Cancer Staging and End-Results Reporting, 1978.

NSABP Protocol 6, a Clinical Trial to Compare Segmental Mastectomy and Axillary Dissection with and without Radiation of the Breast and Total Mastectomy and Axillary Dissection. From NSABP headquarters, University of Philadelphia.

Rosemond, George P. "Pregnancy and Breast Cancer." Chapter 44 in *The Breast,* ed. H. S. Gallager. C. V. Mosby, St. Louis, 1978.

Rosen, Paul P. "The Clinical Significance of Pre-Invasive Breast Carcinoma." *Cancer* 46:919–925, 1980.

Rosen, Paul P. "Predictors of Recurrence in Stage I Breast Carcinoma." *Ann. Surg.,* January 1981.

Rosen, Peter P. "Lobular Carcinoma In Situ of the Breast." *Cancer* 47:813–819, 1981.

Rosenbaum, Ernest. *Decision for Life.* Bull Publishing, Palo Alto, CA, 1980. (Ann described the last years of her life in this book.)

Rosenbaum, Ernest. *Living with Cancer, A Guide for the Patient, the Family, and Friends.* Praeger, 1975.

Rosenbaum, Ernest and Isadora. "Audio Aids in Improving Communication with Patients," paper presented 1981.

Rosenbaum, Ernest and Isadora. *A Comprehensive Guide for Cancer Patients and Their Families.* Bull Publishing, Palo Alto, 1980.

Shapero, Lucy, and Goodman, Anthony. *Never Say Die.* Appleton-Century-Crofts, 1980.

Chapter 7: Restoring the Breast: Reconstruction

Albo R. "Immediate Reconstruction after Modified Mastectomy for Carcinoma of the Breast." *Am. J. Surg.,* July 1980.

Anderson J. "Spread to the Nipple and Areolar in Carcinoma of the Breast." *Ann. Surg.* 189:367, 1979.

Anstice, Elizabeth. "Coping after a Mastectomy." *Nursing Times,* July 9, 1970.

Bostwick, J. "Sixty Latissimus Dorsi Flaps." *Plast. Reconstr. Surg.* 63: 113, 1978.

Bostwick, J. "Breast Reconstruction after Radical Mastectomy." *Plast. Reconstr. Surg.* 61:682, 1978.

Breast Reconstruction, A Woman's Decision. Department of Plastic Surgery, Cleveland Clinic, 1980.

Breast Reconstruction—Creating a New Breast Contour after Mastectomy. NIH Publication No. 81-2151, November 1980.

Breast Reconstruction Following Mastectomy for Cancer—Some Questions and Answers. The American Society of Plastic and Reconstructive Surgeons, Inc., 1979.

Clifford, Edward. "Breast Reconstruction Following Mastectomy: Social Characteristics of Patients Seeking the Procedure" (Part I); "Marital Characteristics of Patients Seeking the Procedure" (Part II). *Ann. Plast. Surg,* November 1980.

Clifford, Edward. "The Reconstruction Experience: The Search for Restitution." In *Breast Reconstruction Following Mastectomy,* ed. N. G. Georgiade. C. V. Mosby, St. Louis, 1979.

Cronin, T. D. "Augmentation Mammoplasty, A New 'Natural Feel' Prosthesis." *Plast. Reconstr. Surg.* 1:46, 1970.

Dicker, Ralph L. *Consultation with a Plastic Surgeon.* Warner Books, 1975.

Dowden, R. V. "Advising the Mastectomy Patient about Reconstruction." *Am. Fam. Physician,* May 1979.

Dowden, R. V. "The Breast Reconstruction Patient and Her Health Insurance Carrier." *JAMA*, Dec. 21, 1979.

Ford, Betty. *The Times of My Life*. Ballantine, 1978.

Gayou, Robert. "Capsular Contracture around Silicone Mammary Prostheses." *Ann. Plast. Surg.*, January 1979.

Goldwyn, Robert. "Vincent Czerny and the Beginnings of Breast Reconstruction." *Plast. Reconstr. Surg.*, May 1978.

Greenberg, Roger. "Breast Reconstruction after Mastectomy." *What's New in Cancer Care*. West Coast Cancer Foundation, July 1980.

Horton, Charles. "Immediate Reconstruction Following Mastectomy for Cancer." *Clin. Plast. Surg.* 6:37, 1979.

LaBarre, Harriet. *Plastic Surgery: Beauty You Can Buy*. Holt, Rinehart and Winston, 1970.

McCraw, John. "Post-Mastectomy Rehabilitation: A Comprehensive Appraisal, Part I: Pre-operative Considerations." Paper presented to American Association of Plastic Surgeons, Scottsdale, AZ, May 14, 1980.

Maxwell, G. Patrick. "Cancer Trends: Breast Reconstruction after Mastectomy." *Va. Med. Mon.*, May 1981.

Maxwell, G. Patrick. "Latissimus Dorsi Breast Reconstruction, an Aesthetic Assessment." *Clin. Plast. Surg.*, April 1981.

Maxwell, G. Patrick. "Post-Mastectomy Rehabilitation: A Comprehensive Appraisal. Part II: Operative Considerations Presented." American Society for Aesthetic Plastic Surgery, Orlando, FL, May 18, 1980.

"Medical Implants: What Can Go Wrong?" *Science News*, April 12, 1980.

Millard, D. Ralph. "Breast Reconstruction after a Radical Mastectomy." *Plast. Reconstr. Surg.*, September 1976.

Rosato, Francis, "Postmastectomy Breast Reconstruction." *Current Problems in Surgery*, vol. 17, no. 11, November 1980 Yearbook Medical Publishers Inc., Chicago.

Shedbalker, A. "A Study of Effects of Radiation on Silicone Prostheses." *Plast. Reconstr. Surg.* 65:805, 1980.

Snyderman, R. K. "Reconstruction of the Female Breast Following Radical Mastectomy." *Plast. Reconstr. Surg.* 47:565, 1971.

Stallings, James O. *A New You*. Signet, 1977.

Thomas, Sally G. "Breast Reconstruction Following Mastectomy." Paper presented at Second International Conference on Oncology Nursing, London, England, Sept. 4, 1980.

Thomas, Sally G. "Confronting One's Changed Image. *Am. J. Nurs.*, September 1977.

Chapter 8: Saving the Breast: Radiation

"Breast Cancer: The Retreat from Radical Surgery." *Consumer Reports*, January 1981.

"Breast Saving Surgery, Radiation for Early Cancer Gaining Advocates." *JAMA*, Feb. 20, 1981.

Calle, R. "Conservative Management of Operable Breast Cancer." *Cancer* 42: 2045, 1978.

Cope, Oliver. *The Breast: Its Problems, Benign and Malignant, and How to Deal with Them.* Houghton Mifflin, Boston, 1978.

Curie, Eve. *Madame Curie.* Doubleday, 1937.

Grobstein, Ruth. Lectures. San Francisco Regional Cancer Foundation program on the State of the Art for Breast Cancer Treatment, March 26, 1981; Women's Center, University of California, Berkeley, April 22, 1981.

Harris, Jay. "Primary Radiation Therapy for Breast Cancer." *Ann. Rev. Med.,* ed. W. P. Creger, vol. 32, pp. 3872–04, Annual Reviews, Inc., Palo Alto, CA. 1981.

Harris, Jay. "The Role of Radiation Therapy in the Primary Treatment of Carcinoma of the Breast." *Semin. Oncol.,* December 1978.

Hellman, Samuel. "Radiation Therapy of Early Carcinoma of the Breast without Mastectomy." *Cancer* 46:988–994, 1980.

Levene, Martin. "Alternative Therapy, A New Role for Radiation Therapy." *Am. J. Nurs.,* September 1977.

Levene, Martin. "Overall Principles of Cancer Management, Radiation." Chapter 8 in *Cancer, a Manual for Practitioners,* Fifth Edition, American Cancer Society, Massachusetts Division, 1978.

Montague, Eleanor. "Radiotherapy as Primary Modality in Treatment of Curable Breast Cancer." Chapter 20 in *The Breast,* ed. H. S. Gallager, C. V. Mosby, St. Louis, 1978.

Mustakallio, S. "Conservative Treatment of Breast Carcinoma, Review of 25 Years Follow Up." *Clin. Radiol.* 23:110–116, 1972.

Peters, M. Vera. "Wedge Resection and Irradiation, an Effective Treatment in Early Breast Cancer." *JAMA,* April 10, 1967.

Radiation Therapy and You—A Guide to Self-Help During Treatment. NIH Publication No. 80-2227, August 1980.

"Radiotherapists Challenge Surgeons on Breast Cancer." *Medical World News,* Nov. 10, 1980.

Ristom, Juliet. Statement made at the hearing of the California State Senate Committee on Business and Professions Code, April 9, 1980.

Veronesi, Umberto. "Value of Limited Surgery for Breast Cancer." *Semin. Oncol.,* December 1978.

Chapter 9: Future Directions

Cancer in California. Reference issue of the *ACS Volunteer,* vol. 27, no. 1, 1981.

Colcher, D. "A Spectrum of Monoclonal Antibodies Reactive with Human Mammary Tumor Cells." *Proc. Nat. Acad. Sci.,* in press.

Dritschilo, Anthony. "Therapeutic Implications of Heat as Related to Radiation Therapy." *Semin. Oncol.,* March 1981.

Grady, Denise. "Shedding Light on the Breast." *Discover,* March 1981.

"Hyperthermia, Still Experimental, May Win Place in Cancer Therapy." *JAMA,* March 20, 1981.

"Interferon Results Still Too Early, Incomplete; Prospects Grow as Clinical Trials Stepped Up." *Clinical Cancer Letter*, March 1980.

"Keeping in Touch—A Breast Self-Examination Teaching Project in Dane County, Wis. High Schools." *Wisconsin Clinical Cancer Center*, June, 1978.

King, Mary-Claire. "Allele Increasing Susceptibility to Human Breast Cancer May Be Linked to the Glutamate-Pyruvate Transaminase Locus." *Science*, April 25, 1980.

Marx, Jean. "Interferon Congress Highlights." *Science*, Nov. 28, 1980.

Milstein, Cesar. "Monoclonal Antibodies." *Scientific America*, October 1980.

Ohlsson, Bjorn. "Diaphanography: A Method for Evaluation of the Female Breast." *World J. Surg.*, 4:701, 1980.

Schlom, Jeffrey. "Generation of Human Monoclonal Antibodies Reactive with Human Mammary Carcinoma Cells." *Proc. Natl. Acad. Sci.*, November 1980.

Terman, David S. "Preliminary Observations of the Effects on Breast Adenocarcinoma of Plasma Perfused over Immobilized Protein A." *New Engl. J. Med.*, Nov. 12, 1981.

Selected Readings

Chapter 2: A Lump: What Does It Mean?

Milan, Albert R. *Breast Self-Examination.* Liberty Publishing Co., paperback, 1980.

Rothenberg, Robert E. *The Complete Book of Breast Care.* Ballantine, paperback, 1975.

Chapter 4: Breast Cancer Psychology

Ayalah, Daphna, and Weinstock, Isaac J. *Breasts: Women Speak About Their Breasts and Their Lives.* Summit Books, paperback, 1979.

Comfort, Alex. *Joy of Sex.* Simon and Schuster, paperback, 1972.

Kaplan, Helen S. *The New Sex Therapy: Active Treatment of Sexual Dysfunction* Times Books, 1974.

McCarthy, Berry W. *What You Still Don't Know About Male Sexuality.* Crowell, 1977.

Sontag, Susan. *Illness As Metaphor.* Random House, paperback, 1977.

Chapter 5: Where Are We Today?

Crile, George. *Surgery, Your Choices and Alternatives.* Delacorte Press, 1970.

Kushner, Rose. *Why Me?* Signet, 1977.

Morra, Marion, and Potts, Eva. *Choices, Realistic Alternatives in Cancer Treatment.* Avon, paperback, 1980.

Chapter 6: It's Cancer—Now What Happens?

Eating Hints: Recipes and Tips for Better Nutrition During Cancer Treatment. U.S. Dept. of Health and Human Services, NIH Pub. No. 80-2079, August 1980. (Available from Office of Cancer Communications, National Cancer Institute, Bethesda, MD 20205.)

Kübler-Ross, Elisabeth. *On Death and Dying.* Macmillan, 1972.

Morra, Marion, and Potts, Eve. *Choices, Realistic Alternatives in Cancer Treatment.* Avon, paperback, 1980.

Rosenbaum, Ernest and Isadora. *A Comprehensive Guide for Cancer Patients and Their Families.* Bull Publishing, Palo Alto, CA, 1980.

Chapter 7: Restoring the Breast: Reconstruction

Zalon, Jean. *I Am Whole Again: The Case for Breast Reconstruction after Mastectomy.* Random House, 1978.

Chapter 8: Saving the Breast: Radiation

Cope, Oliver. *The Breast: Its Problems, Benign and Malignant, and How to Deal with Them.* Houghton Mifflin, 1978.

Cleveland; Peter Kwok, Staff Pharmacist, Alta Bates Hospital Berkeley; Henry Patrick Leis, Jr., Clinical Professor of Surgery, Chief of the Breast Service and Co-

Additional
Acknowledgements

Robert J. Albo, surgeon, Oakland, and Assistant Clinical Professor of Surgery, University of California, San Francisco; Christine A. Freedman, typist; Lonnie Garfield Barbach, sex therapist in private practice and author of *For Yourself* and *Shared Intimacies*; Jan Bowers, Assistant Director of Communications, American College of Radiology; Stephen K. Carter, Director, Northern California Cancer Program; Michael J. Cassidy, Director, Medical Oncology, Alta Bates Hospital, Berkeley; Norman R. Cohen, medical oncologist, Berkeley, and Associate Clinical Professor of Medicine, University of California, San Francisco; Richard J. Cohen, Chief of Oncology, Children's Hospital, San Francisco; Raymond Colvig, Director, Public Information Office, University of California, Berkeley; Oliver Cope, Professor Emeritus of Surgery, Harvard Medical School; Helen Crothers, Service and Rehabilitation Assistant, California Division, American Cancer Society; Vincent T. DeVita, Jr., Director, National Cancer Institute; Melvyn I. Dinner, Chairman, Department of Plastic, Reconstructive, and Aesthetic Surgery, Cleveland Clinic; Richard V. Dowden, Department of Plastic, Reconstructive, and Aesthetic Surgery, Cleveland Clinic; Harold Ellis, Professor, Westminster Medical School, London; Carol Fegte, medical editor; Marcia Kraft Goin, Department of Psychiatry and Behavioral Sciences, University of Southern California School of Medicine; Ruth H. Grobstein, Department of Radiation Therapy, University of California, San Francisco; Adeline Hackett, Director, Peralta Cancer Research Institite, Oakland; Jay R. Harris, Department of Radiation Therapy, Harvard Medical School; Kaye Heinz, founding director, AWEAR; Donald Earl Henson, Chief of Diagnostic Procedures, National Cancer Institute Breast Cancer Task Force; Chuck Honaker, Director of Communications, American College of Radiology; Charles E. Horton, Professor and Chairman, Department of Plastic Surgery, Eastern Virginia Medical School; Thomas K. Hunt, Professor of Surgery, University of California, San Francisco; Philip B. Kivitz, Director, San Francisco Breast Evaluation Center; Janet E. Krejci, RENU Program, director of the Institute of Breast Disease, New York Medical College; Brian J. Lewis, Associate Clinical Professor, University of California, San Francisco; John B. McCraw, Department of Plastic Surgery, Eastern Virginia Medical School; G. Patrick Maxwell, Department of Plastic Surgery, Eastern Virginia Medical School; R. Barrett Noone, Chief of Plastic Surgery, Lankenan Hospital and Bryn Mawr Hospital, Philadelphia; Vincent Pennisi, Director Emeritus, Plastic and Reconstructive Surgery Center, St. Francis Memorial Hospital, San Francisco; Nicholas L. Petrakis, Chairman, Department of Epidemiology and International Health, University of California, San Francisco; Theodore R. Purcell, Director of Radiation Oncology, Alta Bates Hospital, Berkeley; Ernest H. Rosenbaum, Associate Chief of Medicine, Mount Zion Hospital and Medical Center, San Francisco; Isadora R. Rosenbaum, Medical Assistant in Oncology, Mount Zion Hospital and Medical Center, San Francisco; Otto W. Sartorius, Surgeon, Santa Barbara; Wendy S. Schain, Medical Health Consultant, National Institutes of Health; Laszlo Tabar, Director, Mammography Department, Falun Hospital, Falun, Sweden; Sally Galbraith Thomas, Associate Professor, School of Nursing, University of California, Los Angeles; Luis O. Vasconez, Chief, Division of Plastic Surgery, University of California, San Francisco; Umberto Veronesi, Director, National Cancer Institute, Milan, Italy; Farrell Wolfson, Office of Cancer Communication, National Cancer Institute; Bernie Zilbergeld, sex therapist in private practice and author of *Male Sexuality*

Finally, I wish to thank those who helped make publication of this book possible: author and journalist Lacey Fosburgh, my agent, Patricia Berens, and her assistant, Cynthia Manson, of the Sterling Lord Agency, and my editor, Marie Cantlon.

I would appreciate receiving comments from readers, in care of Beacon Press.

Index

Mary J. Spletter, a science writer who specializes in public health, cancer research, psychology, and sociology, works at the Office of Public Information, University of California, Berkeley. An active volunteer in the American Cancer Society's Reach-to-Recovery program where she counsels women who have undergone mastectomies, she travels widely to speak about her personal experiences with cancer and breast reconstruction.